Dementia: A Positive Response

Hope, Help and Humour on the Journey

Dr William A. M. Cutting

Onwards and Upwards Publishers

3 Radfords Turf, Cranbrook, Exeter, EX5 7DX, United Kingdom.

www.onwardsandupwards.org

Published in the United Kingdom by Onwards and Upwards Publishers (2018).

ISBN:	978-1-78815-675-2
Typeface:	Sabon LT
Illustrator:	Ann Marsden
Graphic design:	LM Graphic Design

Printed in the United Kingdom.

About the Author

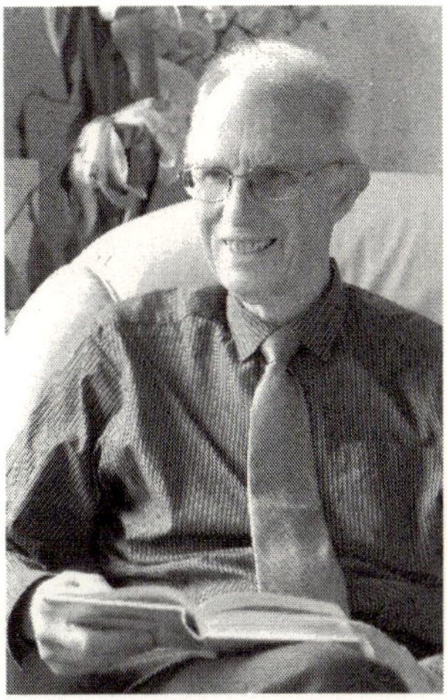

William Cutting was born in South India where his father was a medical missionary. He trained in medicine at the University of Edinburgh where he met his wife, Margot, who was also training for medical mission work. They worked in rural India, Andhra Pradesh, for twelve years, developing simple child health services and using nutrition rehabilitation to help mothers feed their malnourished children back to health with local foods.

After six years at the London School of Hygiene and Tropical Medicine and the Tropical Child Health Unit of the Institute of Child Health, Great Ormond Street, Dr Cutting was appointed to the Department of Child Life and Health of the University of Edinburgh with special responsibility for international paediatric trainees. He also acted as consultant with WHO, UNICEF, British Council etc.

Cutting's research interests were wide. At one time he was responsible for two small international teams. In Bangladesh they studied zinc supplementation and catch-up growth in malnourished children, and in Zaire (now the Democratic Republic of Congo), HIV infection in children. Through his work he gained much interesting international experience, many contacts and friends.

After retiring in 1998, Dr Cutting's wide clinical and pastoral interests turned to the many and varied needs of the elderly. He started to collect material, write for and befriend a circle of older people. The paediatrician metamorphosed into a concerned amateur geriatrician.

Endorsements

William Cutting's book is superb, positive and covers just about every aspect of dementia in a way that is easily understood. It is interspersed with delightful drawings, amusing pieces and personal stories. He has also drawn together much that is helpful from many other sources. This book should be a great encouragement and valuable resource for many.

Dr. Jennifer Bute
Former GP and founder of Glorious Opportunity website, after she was diagnosed with dementia, to support others living with dementia

Being diagnosed with dementia is surely always devastating and increasingly life-changing. However, 'Dementia: A Positive Response' demonstrates clearly that all is not total darkness. In this easy-to-read book, we learn (perhaps surprisingly) that there can be positives for both victim and carer – including ways in which we can reduce the likelihood of developing dementia or slowing its progress.

Further, we are reminded that a Christian perspective gives an added dimension: "...even if much of the brain has been destroyed, the soul remains. The real person is still there, fully remembered, known to and deeply loved by God, and worthy of care and respect." And those last five words provide the basis for the individual person-centred supportive care championed throughout the book. Strongly recommended.

Dr Robert Twycross (FRCP)
Emeritus Clinical Reader in Palliative Medicine
Oxford University

This delightful book of analysis, anecdote and comic insights is a welcome antidote to the pessimism that dominates so much commentary on the contemporary scourge of dementia. As a practising lawyer and a priest, I only wish William Cutting's book had been available when I was training in each profession. I commend it for careful study by students and practitioners in both – and by everyone with an interest in human development and decline.

Canon John Rees
Legal Adviser to the Archbishop of Canterbury

'Dementia, A Positive Response' is an up-to-date summary and condensation of the help available for people with dementia and those who care about and for them.

William really achieves what it says in its subtitle, providing "hope, help and humour" about one of the growing challenges of our 21st century. He comes at it from the angle of a life-long medical man, a paediatrician but also a carer. It helped me to have known William and his wife Margot for many years.

It is a varied, comprehensive, sympathetic and realistic handbook. It is not a book to be read through, but [rather] dipped into for the information we need when we or others we know face this illness. He has made the contents accessible, professional and readable by carers and patients alike. It will be a great 'find' to very many people in their time of need.

Rev. Tom Houston
Retired after international Christian ministry, leadership and experience as a personal carer

William Cutting has done it again – another wonderful book on growing old, full of information, sensitive humour, wise advice and spiritual understanding.

This time he helps us face dementia, something that will come close to nearly all of us at some time – whether in the family, in friends or in ourselves. It is a book I want on my bookshelf, so as to be able to consult it, to lend it and to recommend it warmly to others.

Rev. David Wenham

New Testament scholar and teacher in India, Bristol and Oxford.

This is the most inspiring and helpful book on dementia that I have read. For those concerned that their forgetfulness is an early sign of this illness, for those needing practical help in living with dementia, for carers, especially those on the edge of burnout, for Christians who feel God has abandoned them in this illness and for churches and communities wanting to offer a dementia-friendly environment and appropriate pastoral care, reading and learning from this book will be invaluable.

This book is written with clarity, deep insight and understanding, Christian love and a good dose of humour. Dementia touches us all in one way or another on our journey through life so get reading!

Dr Gareth Tuckwell

Retired hospice medical director and chairman of Sanctuary Care (which provides a home for thousands with dementia)

In the face of the global challenge of Alzheimer's disease to both health and social care, Dr Cutting's book is a very positive and practical response. It not only addresses the needs of those with this dreadful condition, but also the great demands on the carers, who often suffer with the patients.

The book highlights the importance of simple things; the loving touch, music, smiles and laughter. He and I believe that a sense of humour is part of the human personality and laughter is a divine gift. In this practical book on a most serious illness, the therapy benefits from the injection of pages of comic relief.

A man of Christian faith, Dr Cutting points out that though dementia can rob a person of both brain and body, it cannot steal the soul.

If you know someone caring for a person with dementia, sell your shirt if need be, buy and give this book. It will be a double blessing.

The Very Rev. Dr. James Simpson

Former Moderator of the General Assembly of the Church of Scotland and Minister of Dornoch Cathedral

Acknowledgements

Thanks – to family and friends, in particular to three men: *Archie Dale, Peter Little* and *John Blackie.* Archie and Peter encouraged me to share what I had learnt about dementia from my own perspective. Archie was an exemplary primary carer for his own wife, Margaret, with dementia. With help from his daughter and one other carer he gave her all the personal care in an exceptional manner, in their own home, right up to her death. He loaned me his large collection of books and gave me countless practical suggestions.

Some of Peter's relatives and friends had been helped by my *Face the Future* book series and so he was keen that I should complete this book too. He read the proofs and made many valuable comments. John has, on several occasions, rescued me from problems with my computer that were blocking progress. Thank you all three.

Thanks also – to two important ladies. *Ann Marsden*, who was a former colleague in India, freely gave her time, artistic skills and quiet humour to illustrate the book. Also *Louise Morse*, who is an expert in dementia, an inspiring speaker and a well-known author, generously shared information, advised, encouraged and wrote the Foreword.

Thanks also to a number of authors who have allowed me to quote from their books and papers, and use their photographs.

Finally I am very grateful for the guidance and help from *Luke Jeffery,* Director at Onwards and Upwards Publishers.

To my wife Margot.

She not only supported me so faithfully and did a great job bringing up our children, but when diagnosed with dementia in 2014, faced the condition with honesty, faith, composure and quiet courage. She has continued to live life as normally and as fully as possible and is the inspiration for this book.

Contents

Foreword by Louise Morse

Thirteen years ago, when I began researching and gathering materials for my first book, *Could it be Dementia,*[1] the dread of dementia was said to be equal to that of cancer twenty years earlier. Now discoveries have revolutionised treatment to the point that some cancers can be cured and some held at bay during the person's lifetime. A friend in his seventies told me recently that his doctor informed him that although he has leukaemia, he will die *with* it, not *because of* it.

That stage hasn't yet been reached with dementia. There is still no cure because, apart from brain damage following stroke (vascular dementia), the causes are still a mystery. The few available pharmaceuticals only help around one in three people. But encouragingly, rates of dementia diagnoses are dropping all over the world, due, it is thought, to better lifestyles and education. There is not going to be a dementia tsunami, although numbers are projected to rise because people are living much longer and dementia is largely (but not exclusively) a disease of old age.

There will be a breakthrough sooner or later. All over the world scientists are tackling it from different angles. Earlier this year the Alzheimer's Society announced that it was shifting its research focus from the Amyloid B hypothesis as it had failed to produce an effective treatment in over twenty years. The wonder is that the hypothesis was held as the gold standard for so long when other studies, some quite large, had shown that people with extensive brain pathology could have no symptoms of dementia,

---

[1] Louise Morse and Roger Hitchings; *Could It Be Dementia?: Losing Your Mind Doesn't Mean Losing Your Soul;* Monarch (2008); ISBN 9781854248251.

and vice versa. The nuns study,[2] for example, began in 1986 and is still continuing. An interesting finding of this study was that an examination of the essays written by novices in the application stage showed that only 10% of those with good word density developed dementia, which seems to echo current observations about the importance of learning and education to brain health. However, the fact is that people with good levels of education do develop dementia. The mystery remains – why? The trailblazer in understanding dementia, Professor Tom Kitwood of Bradford University, pointed out that our brains' ability to resist dementia may be due to "the degree to which our individual nerve architecture has developed as a result of learning and experience"[3]. A growing body of research points to the importance of psychological wellbeing during our lifetimes. As the Bible says, "Guard your heart with all diligence, for from it flow all of life's consequences."[4]

When I started writing *Could it be...* family doctors were being castigated by the Minister of Health for having "nihilistic" attitudes inhibiting them from making dementia diagnoses. The official government theme became louder and louder: people should be diagnosed with dementia so that they could receive tailored treatment and support. Then, late 2015, a national survey of doctors by the Royal College of GPs found that across 70% of the country there was little, if any, tailored care and support. Rural and semi-rural areas fared best; large conurbations struggled. With cuts in funding for social care, the situation seems little better today.

The best treatment for people with dementia is the quality of the care they receive. Families and caregivers are strengthened and encouraged by knowing as much as possible about the condition. Dr Cutting quotes clinical psychologist Oliver James' statement in

---

[2] Negash S. et al.; *Resilient brain aging: characterization of discordance between Alzheimer's disease pathology and cognition;* Curr Alzheimer Res. (Oct 2013);10(8):844-51; *www.ncbi.nlm.nihgov/pubmed/23919768*

[3] Kitwood; *Dementia Reconsidered* (2002).

[4] Proverbs 4:23 (CJB).

his introduction to James' book, *Contented Dementia*, that "it truly is possible to create wellbeing for the rest of the person's life"[5].

You will read here of Dr Cutting's impressive medical background and his professional history. But when dementia strikes home, as it did with his wife's diagnosis, it becomes a matter of the heart as much as the head. As well as adding to the bank of knowledge about the condition itself, in easy-to-understand, bite-sized chunks, the book lifts the heart with its stories and nuggets of humour. Dr Cutting draws from a range of publications, and distils real life stories written by people whose lives have been impacted by dementia. And, as in the books of his *Face the Future* series, he infuses the pages with compassion and humour. One day, there will be a dementia cure or a preventative – perhaps both. Until then we need to be strengthened mentally, emotionally and spiritually, and you will find much practical help in these pages.

Louise Morse
Author, Cognitive Therapist and
Head of Communications, Pilgrims' Friend Society, U.K.

e. *louise.morse@pilgrimsfriend.org.uk*
t. 0300 3031431
m. 07585 539539

[5] Oliver James; *Contented Dementia?* Vermilion, Ebony Publishing (2008).

PREFACE

How the Book Came to Be Written and Its Objective

For many people, old age creeps up on you when you are busy with other things, and very few of us admit to being old. However, 'old age is not for wimps'; it brings with it a package of problems that we have to face, live with and adjust to: reduced mobility, failing health, 'forgetfulness', a loss of independence, bereavement and loneliness.

But there is much that can be done to face the future in a positive manner.

The French philosopher, Louis-Vincent Thomas said:

> *...only through love, faith and humour can we confront and perhaps transform the terrible realities of old age, decrepitude, and death.*[6]

To combat 'the spectre of old age' in a positive way, I, a former paediatrician, embraced this powerful triumvirate of forces – love, faith and humour – and added practical information. I collected stories, biographic glimpses, poems, jokes

---

[6] Louis-Vincent Thomas quoted by Marie de Hennezel; *The Warmth of the Heart prevents your Body from Rusting;* chapter 1, page 13; Rodale, a division of Macmillan (2011).

and devotionals and wove them into books of practical encouragement for Seniors: the *Face the Future* book series.[7]

Dementia was a topic I knew I must cover. The condition was attacking many of those I was trying to help. It struck friends and the spouses of friends. Some lent me books and one friend was a wonderful caring role-model. Finally the disease stepped into our home, and in 2014 my dear wife was confirmed to have signs of early dementia. As I mentioned in my dedication, she has faced this with honesty, faith, composure and quiet courage.

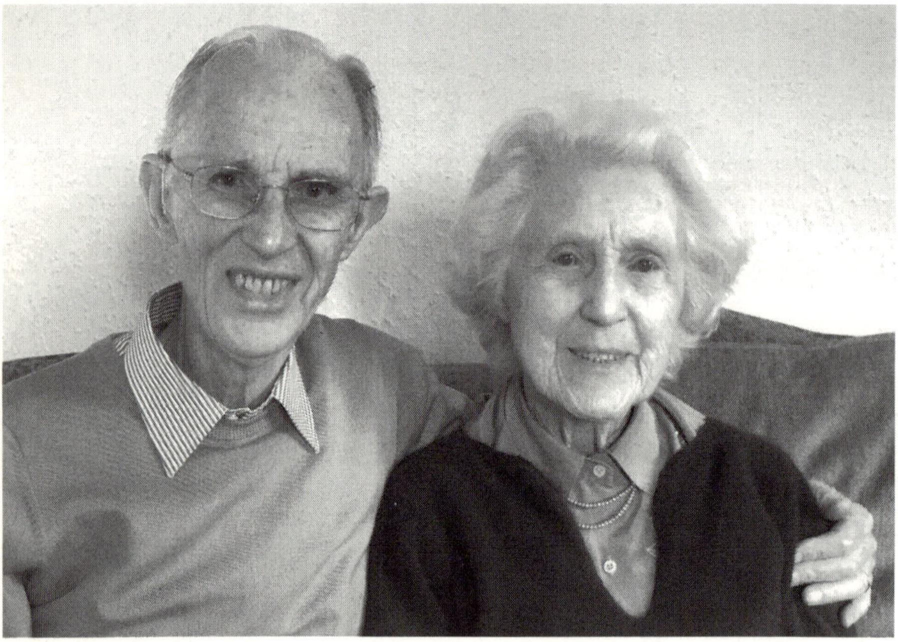

William and Margot Cutting.

---

[7] The books in the *Face the Future* series are:
Seniors can inspire, apply wisdom and model values; Onwards and Upwards (2014); ISBN 978-1-907509-97-1;
Challenges, joy and faith for Seniors; Onwards and Upwards (2014); ISBN 978-1-910197-11-0;
Seniors, make the most of the health you have; Onwards and Upwards (2015); ISBN 978-1-910197-13-4;
Face the Future 4 (not yet published).

My study then went to a deeper level and I realised that dementia demanded a book in its own right. As our lives began a gradual rearrangement of activities and duties, we had our own experience to share. I recognise that although the pathophysiology of the condition is not fully understood and there is no specific or proven medicinal cure, there is so much that can and should be done to help and care.

> The objective of this book is to help those living with dementia, and the families and carers who support them, to live a full, positive and even a comfortable life.

Because the book addresses those with early dementia, and also their families and carers, it sometimes talks directly to those with the condition, but most sections are directed more to the families and carers.

Find here, then, stories that inspire, many practical ideas, a little fun and some divine inspiration from those who have travelled this road.

William A.M. Cutting, MBChB (Edin), FRCPE, FRCPCH

CHAPTER ONE

Introduction to Dementia

> *Dementia is likely to be the health problem that affects us all in the coming decades, especially Seniors, those of us who are older. This is a devastating brain disease. The causes and how it damages function are not fully understood and we have no specific treatment to cure it.*
> *I believe medical science will answer these questions. But for now, we must use the information, the tools and the help we have to live positively with this serious condition.*

Understanding dementia

Dementia is the most serious, devastating and dreaded disease that we all face. It affects the brain and through that incredible organ it can affect almost every component of life. Despite this, from the very outset, be assured that there are reasons for hope!

You may not develop the condition, but it will certainly affect people you know and often people who are close to you. It can affect the most brilliant brains and the most loving and capable family members. Dementia can be the most distressing experience of life. The emotional, psychological, physical and financial cost is beyond calculation.

As Sally Magnusson says in the subtitle of her book,[8] "dementia changes everything".

However it is not all doom and gloom. There may be years – even very many years – of interesting and companionable life, even comfortable and enjoyable life, to be lived on that journey. My wife and I are on that journey and we are determined to make the most of it – and so can you.

> *Seniors, understand dementia and accept its importance, but take courage; you can travel with hope!*

In the introduction to his book *Contented Dementia*, Oliver James states that "however advanced the illness, the real person who means so much to you is still there, ... a great deal of the mind and the emotional self of the person with dementia is still functioning"[9].

Louise Morse, another expert who has written widely on dementia, puts it, "You may lose your brain, but you cannot lose your soul."[10]

Those with dementia need and deserve much personal loving care! In the following pages I have collected practical advice about how best to provide good and appropriate care. Whether you are someone with dementia, a personal carer or someone with a concern about the condition, I want to share reasons for hope and positive encouragement.

---

8 Sally Magnusson; *Mamie. Where Memories Go –Why dementia changes everything;* Two Roads, Hodder & Stoughton (2014).

9 Oliver James; *Contented Dementia;* Vermilion, Ebony Publishing (2008). See chapter 7.

10 Louise Morse and Roger Hitchings; *Could It Be Dementia?: Losing Your Mind Doesn't Mean Losing Your Soul;* Monarch (2008); ISBN 9781854248251.
Louise Morse; *Dementia: Frank and Linda's Story;* Monarch Books (2010).
Louise Morse; *Dementia: Pathways to Hope: Spiritual insights and practical advice;* Monarch Books (2015); ISBN 978-0-85721-655-7.

If you have not yet been affected by this disease in a family member or a close friend, and if you are over sixty years old, it will not be long before it touches you.

THE STATISTICS ABOUT DEMENTIA

> *Dementia is the greatest global challenge for health and social care in the 21st century: around 50 million people worldwide have dementia and this number is predicted to triple by 2050.*[11]

But the statistics are confusing. The proportion of older people in the world, and in Britain in particular, is rising steadily and age is associated with dementia.

In Britain, between the ages of 70 and 79, 1 in 25 people have dementia. It affects 1 in 6 between 80 and 89, and 1 in 3 of those over 90. This is a very steep rise with age!

The bad news. There are now more people with dementia than there have ever been, but that is because there are now more old people still living than there have ever been. Consequently, the prevalence of dementia is greater. Another confusing factor: "Dementia" appears on death certificates more often now than in the past. This is because it is now recognised and accepted as an important cause and contributor to death. It is not that dementia has become a more fatal disease.

The good news. In fact, both in Britain and in North America, the proportion of old people with dementia is now less than it was 20 years ago. The incidence rate (that is, the number of new cases per 1000 population) in each age band is less than it was 10 years earlier.

The reason for this is also good news. People are living longer, receiving better healthcare and making better, healthier lifestyle choices: less smoking, more exercise and a better diet. Professor Carol Brayne, Director of the Cambridge University Institute of

---

[11] Lancet symposium, *Prevention and management of dementia: a priority for public health;* July 2017. *http://dx.doi.org/10.1016/S0140-6736(17)31363-6*

Public Health, says, "Our findings suggest that brain health is improving significantly in the UK across generations, particularly among men."[12]

This means there are things that we can do to delay the onset of dementia and perhaps stop it happening.[13] Estimates of a so-called "dementia 'tsunami'" that might hit Britain could be reduced if appropriate preventive measures are taken.

Although many more people now know about dementia, and there are more patients, many are not diagnosed and therefore not treated appropriately. According to the Alzheimer's Society, in 2014 only 44% of people in England with dementia received a diagnosis.

In 2014 over 850,000 people had dementia in UK. It was estimated that by 2051 the number may exceed 2 million. However, the latest figures on incidence rates and the possibility of preventive programmes will hopefully mean that these projections may be reduced.

This is a worldwide problem, not simply a developed country problem. All countries which have an increasing proportion of people in the 'Senior' age group will have a growing problem with dementia.

WHO PROVIDES CARE AND WHO PAYS?

Two thirds of people with dementia in Britain live in the community, while one third live in a care home.

The estimated cost of caring for one dementia patient in UK who cannot look after himself/herself is £27,600 per year (2015). The equivalent cost of caring for one cancer patient is £6,000 and for a heart disease patient is £3,455. The main reason for this is that with cancer and heart conditions, the treatment may be very

---

[12] Matthews F.E. et al.; *A two decade comparison of incidence of dementia in individuals aged 65 years and older from three geographical areas of England: results of the Cognitive Function Ageing Study I and II;* Nature Communications (19 April 2016); DOI 10.1038/ncomms11398.

[13] See chapter 11.

expensive but the costly part is for only a shorter period. For dementia, care is needed 365 days every year.

In Britain in 2015 dementia was costing the country £26.3 billion per year. Two thirds of the cost of dementia (£17.4 billion) is paid by people with dementia and their families, either in unpaid care (£11.6 billion) or in paying for private social care.

DEMENTIA IS A PERSONAL PROBLEM

The numbers are frightening, but above all else, let us remember that every individual with this dreadful condition is not a statistic but a person; a spouse, a brother, a friend, a mother or a granddad. Clothe every number with skin and give them the face and name of a real person. Each one of them needs much love and appropriate care and so does their distressed family. For this reason, the pattern of the book starts with the personal stories of four individual people: Muriel, Bonnie, Mamie and Jennifer.

We will hear Frank and Linda's story through the words of Louise Morse.[14] It describes the journey of Frank's early dementia in some detail. We can see how they coped with the condition. There follows a review of the features of the condition and then many interventions and strategies that can be used to help those with dementia and those who are helping them. This includes a Christian response to this disease and the assurance that the God who is especially concerned for the vulnerable will never forget those with this dreaded disease, even though they may feel lost and alone. Finally in this section is advice on how best to care for those with challenging behaviours in advanced disease.

From the stories about those with dementia it is sad to see how the disease completely changed their lives, and also the lives of those closest to them. But also inspiring is how their nearest and dearest coped and made the new relationships something of beauty from the tragedy.

---

[14] See page 39.

Response to dementia

The dementia scenario is alarming, but there is much that can and should be done on an individual, a local, a national and even an international level. Many activities will be indicated in the following sections. These include:

- Prevent the disease and slow its progress by attention to the known risk factors. Many things can be done.
- Diagnose more promptly.
- Give better care – social, mental, physical and spiritual. Stimulation can maintain function and enhance and prolong positive life experience.
- Educate the public about prevention and management, and train and support carers, many of whom are family members and the public.
- Support research into causes, prevention and treatment.

The response to dementia should not just be alarm, but action, help and hope!

In Lighter Mode

If humour is kindly, softly meant, not personal or offensive, it is truly a tonic.

There is no more serious subject than dementia. But even in the direst of situations it is essential to retain a sense of humour.

There is certainly no intention to laugh *at* those with dementia, but sometimes it is good to laugh *with* them at some of life's situations...

There is no medication like laughter. For this reason, this serious book deliberately contains some lighthearted passages and some corny jokes. These sections are indicated by the heading 'In Lighter Mode'.

Laughter is the best therapy for the widest range of conditions, but, like the benefits of the sunshine after a dull, distressing day, it has never been subjected to a controlled clinical trial. However, the most miserable patient and the dullest physician agree that laughter works wonders.

Always laugh when you can, it is cheap medicine.

George Gordon Byron

With mirth and laughter let old wrinkles come.

William Shakespeare, The Merchant of Venice

You don't stop laughing because you grow old.
You grow old because you stop laughing.

Michael Pritchard

Worry is the secret weapon of the dark forces of the world that lurk in fear, uncertainty, confusion, stress and loss.
On the other hand, we have our own secret weapon against these fiends. It is laughter.

Vera Nazarian, The Perpetual Calendar of Inspiration

If we couldn't laugh we would all go insane.

Robert Frost

CHAPTER TWO

Dementia: Personal Stories, Real People

This chapter starts with the real life experience of four people with dementia. There are three love stories, descriptions of the devastation that dementia caused, but they also demonstrate love's response in three families. The final story is about Dr Jennifer Bute. Amazingly, she challenged the monster and transformed it to be a "glorious opportunity" to help other people come to terms with the condition. What a magnificent role-model she is and what practical hope she dispenses!

Dementia is always about people, and the response should always be love and care. Here are glimpses from the lives of Muriel, Bonnie, Mamie and Jennifer. The first three are vignettes, brief accounts, a glimpse of a life and a profound love, the love of a husband for a wife or a daughter for her mother. Each story, condensed from a book, tells of a vibrant and vital life that was slowly and sadly stolen away, step by step, by dementia, that dreadful, progressive, irreversible disease of the brain. But in each story, a deep response of love was evoked that bore fruit in practical caring and determination to do something about the devastating disease.

Each story is different, but all share the grim, gradual pattern of confusion, fear, anguish, helplessness and loss. It is the agonising loss of a person who has loved and cared for you progressively drifting away so they no longer know you and cannot care for you or care for themselves. Ultimately, it is the deep sorrow of a living death, the demise of a beloved personality months or years before their physical death.

Nothing can adequately prepare a spouse, a child or a family carer for the psychological trauma and the increasing demands that leave the body exhausted, the spirit devastated and the bank account plundered.

Each story is a cry of anguish, yet shining through each is a devotion and a vitality of spirit to make the most of the shreds of life, a passion to pour out loving care and a determination to share the experience so that others may look forward positively with some hope in their hearts.

Muriel McQuilkin

A PROMISE KEPT – THE STORY OF AN UNFORGETTABLE LOVE[15]

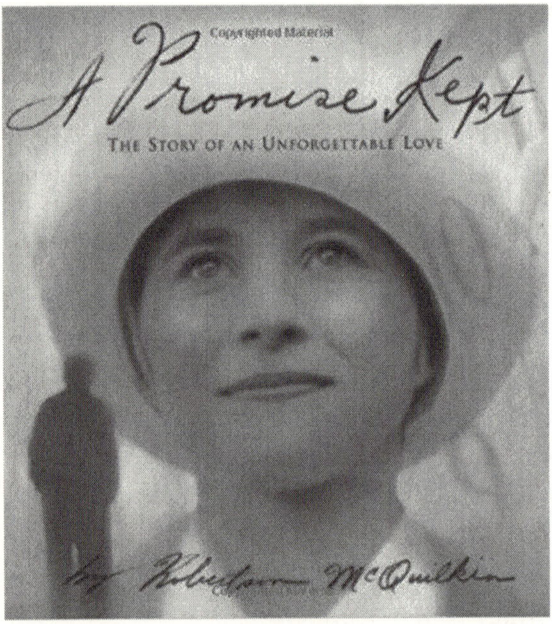

A Promise Kept.

[15] Robertson McQuilkin; Tyndale House Publishers Inc. (1998).

Life is Simpler, Now
Part of a poem written by Robertson McQuilkin.

Life is simpler, now;
Defined no longer
By what we do
So much as who we are:
I am your security,
My companionship
Your only haven
From the buffeting of
Strange winds
Deeply felt
And little understood;
I am set to shield you
From those grim terrors
That may lurk around the bend,

And you?
Your mind is tethered
By strands of love
And joy and tough endurance,
Woven strong across the years.
Hammered by the blows
Of adverse winds.
Love more pure, intense,
Emerges from the fire.

Life is simpler, now –
God's good gift
For two busy people
Who celebrate the past
And patiently wait with hope.

Muriel McQuilkin, was the talented 55-year-old wife of Robertson, the President of Columbia Seminary in USA (1968-1990). She was a conference speaker in her own right and had her own radio and TV programmes. When Alzheimer's disease struck, she was quickly taken off the air, but for some time she still had confidence and curiosity and would often wander and get lost. Many aspects of her behaviour became bizarre, but her devotion to, dependence on and love for her husband deepened as other contacts fell away. Robertson gave up his many local and international responsibilities to care for her full-time. Reflecting on his changed responsibilities, he handed the matter to God: "Father, no regrets, I like this different assignment." God blessed him with his divine approval of his new, simpler caring role.

Muriel did not die until over twenty years after diagnosis, and was personally cared for all the way by her husband. After her passing he was often asked, "How are you doing?" He never mentioned relief but said he was "grieving with gratitude"; gratitude for many great memories, and gratitude that he was able to outlive her, care for her and love her to her last breath.

Bonnie Suchet

MY BONNIE – HOW DEMENTIA STOLE THE LOVE OF MY LIFE[16]

John Suchet is an internationally famous news reporter who won a television lifetime achievement award for investigative journalism, courageous reporting from war zones and professional newscasting. He saw action in the Iran revolution, Northern Ireland at the height of the troubles and the Russian invasion of Afghanistan. On one occasion, he and his camera crew, dressed as Mujahidins, found themselves in front of a Russian firing squad.

His romance with, and marriage to, American beauty queen Bonnie, who had been educated at Cornell University in New

[16] John Suchet; Harper Collins (2010).

York State, could make a Hollywood drama. Their complementary personalities and mutual support were remarkable. While John became an ITV news-reading legend, for 15 years she was the dedicated and efficient London PA to an Irish-American millionaire whose ambition in life was to endow educational enterprises worldwide.[17]

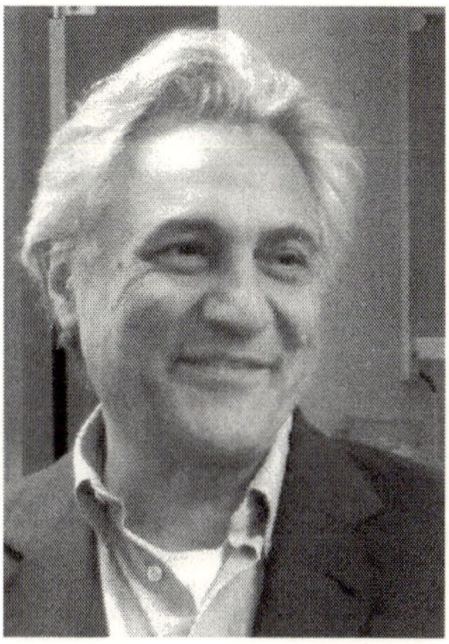

John Suchet. International journalist, newscaster and music presenter.

Bonnie's first signs of Alzheimer's disease, in her early sixties, were simply forgetting things and losing her way. But inexorably it progressed. She was still there, but she wasn't. There were times of apathy and sometimes irrational and obsessional behaviour. John lost his loving, competent, dynamic wife and companion. Progressively he had to take over doing everything. It was exhausting, frustrating and lonely. John's tears and tantrums were followed by guilt and dark despair.

At this desperate time, Ian Weatherhead, from the Admiral Nurses of Dementia UK,[18] came into their life with much wise counsel and practical help. Over many months Ian was able to

[17] John Suchet; *My Bonnie – How dementia stole the love of my life;* Harper Collins (2010).

[18] Admiral Nurses; Dementia UK, 356 Holloway Road (Second Floor), London N7 6PA; tel: (0207) 6974160; *info@dementiauk.org*

explain what was happening to them both and gave strategies to help John cope. John said, “It is not an exaggeration to say that Ian saved my life.” He had to come to terms with the fact that over a couple of years his life had drastically changed; from being Bonnie’s husband and lover, he had become her carer, nurse and home help.

In February 2009, John Suchet, international news reporter and TV celebrity, spoke in a series of interviews on the media. This master of television interrogation had to describe the heart-break of having to care personally for his beloved wife with this dreadful disease. It was emotionally draining, but his words and tears had a powerful impact on the British public. The reality and horror of dementia hit the national consciousness. It was also a massive boost to tens of thousands of carers whose loving labour for those with the disease was frequently overlooked. As never before, John and Bonnie’s tragedy recognised, appreciated and encouraged the role of countless carers and highlighted their need for support. That was a great legacy!

Mamie Baird

WHERE MEMORIES GO – WHY DEMENTIA CHANGES EVERYTHING[19]

This is a deeply moving love story of children for a wonderful and talented mother. It is told by Sally, the eldest child of journalists Magnus Magnusson and Mamie Baird. Mamie was a brilliant woman and a remarkable personality. Sally herself is an award-winning journalist, a TV presenter and an anchor of Reporting Scotland. She honestly and intimately exposes her own, and the family’s, painful experience. The unifying theme of the narrative is the tribute to her wonderful and gifted mother, and the growing anguish as her brilliant brain, imagination and memory were first pilfered and then plundered by this dreadful

[19] Sally Magnusson; Two Roads, Hodder & Stoughton (2014).

disease. It is painful to see in detail the parent/child role reversal that the disease demanded.

The purpose of telling the harrowing story is not any desire for exhibitionism, but it is a cry from the heart. Sally professionally probes the scientific basis of this horrible disease and she lucidly simplifies the current medical understanding of the disorder. She explains the roots of some of the scientific terms used and gives a brief account of some of the personalities who have studied the condition. She makes a frank exposé of the hopeless inadequacy of the British medical and social systems to provide the right quality and quantity of care needed for those with this tragic condition. (To be fair, some people have had a much better experience of the medical and social care systems in UK.)

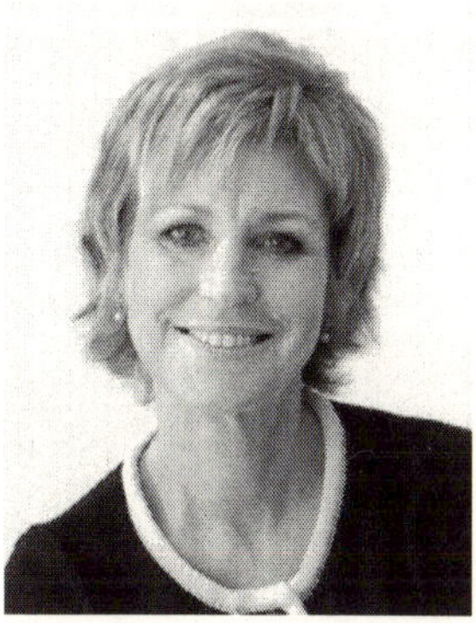

Sally Magnusson, TV newscaster, presenter, author and dementia campaigner.

Sally clearly identifies and specifies several key requirements for a good dementia service: dedicated leadership, a culture of compassion, specific understanding of the condition which requires training and continuity of care. The family found that these components are difficult to find, hard to cultivate and costly in both the private and public sectors.

Sally makes some positive practical suggestions. Despite Mamie's limited ability to respond, the family found and adapted some ways to improve the quality of care. When words fail, two techniques of communication that proved of value were touch and music. Fear is less frightening when you hold hands. Grief can be eased with an appropriate hug and kiss. What a depth of practical agape love the Magnusson sisters demonstrated.

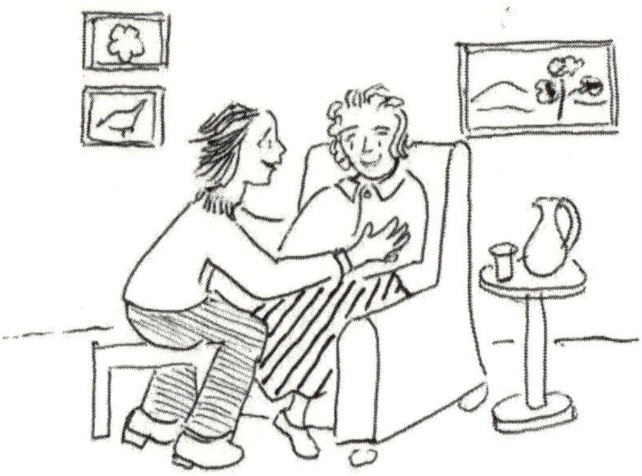

Compassion and love, a warm hug and a kiss can bypass brain blockage!

Then music, especially personal, meaningful music, seems able to transcend or bypass the pathologically blocked pathways of communication. Sally has started a charity, Playlist For Life, that encourages everyone with dementia to have a personal digital collection of favourite music from their early life. Its vision is "that every person with dementia has access to a unique playlist of their life, to help unlock who they are".

Go to *www.playlistforlife.org.uk* on the Internet and you will be helped to set up such a list. There you will also see amazing videos showing the remarkable results when those with dementia hear 'their songs', sing along and smile again.

After losing her mother to dementia, Sally declared, "I hate this disease with a boiling fury," and she is campaigning to do something about it. In an interview in 2014, Sally was pleading for action, research and better care for those with dementia.

> *It's my generation and the one after that needs to look at this and find solutions instead of just being obsessed with being youthful for as long as possible.*[20]

Every person concerned for the wellbeing of Seniors should join in this campaign.

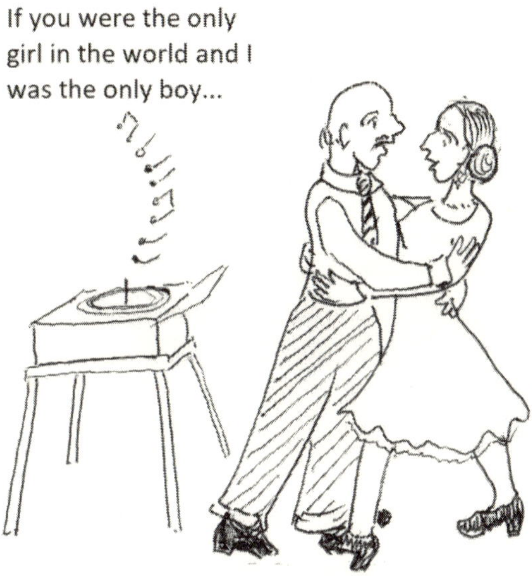
If you were the only girl in the world and I was the only boy...

Some people who have been mute for many months can be revitalised by their favourite music.

Dr Jennifer Bute

GLORIOUS OPPORTUNITY

Dr Jennifer Bute's story is inspiring, making the best of the situation for the sake of others: "How to live with zest for the time you have left!"

Jennifer Bute was a very competent and caring doctor from a leading London medical college. After five training jobs in Britain, with plenty of practical experience under her belt, she worked in

---

[20] Sally Magnusson; *Mamie. Where Memories Go – Why dementia changes everything;* Two Roads, Hodder & Stoughton (2014).

an isolated Christian hospital in Zululand in Southern Africa. Then she returned to UK, married, had three children and worked in a General Practice for 25 years. She was highly respected in her professional work and regarded as a role-model in her community.

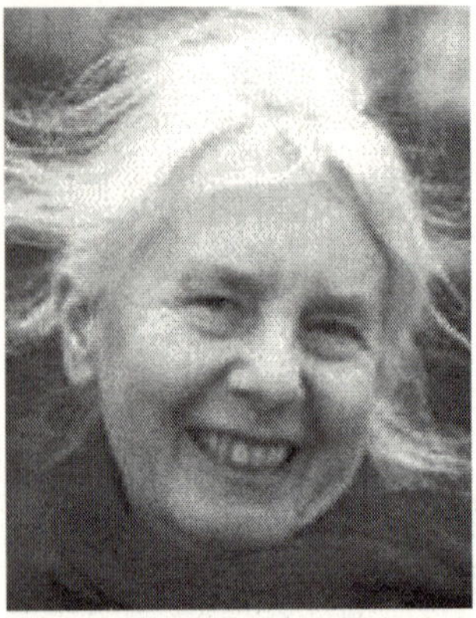

Jennifer Bute, general practitioner, medical missionary, mother and dementia activist living with dementia.

Then a few unexpected things started to happen. She had a 'turn' that was called a TIA (Transient Ischaemic Attack) believed to be due to a brief time of poor blood supply to part of her brain. She also noticed that she would lose her way around roads she knew well, and one day she became confused in the local supermarket. To avoid making mistakes in her work, she became obsessional, taking down notes and answering letters and e-mails by return. Her strategies for coping with forgetfulness helped her to appear normal when she was struggling. Then one day when she was chairing a medical meeting, she could not recognise the people around her, some of whom had been colleagues for many years. It was a defining moment.

Two neurology specialists declared that there was nothing wrong with her. She felt humiliated when one of them told her she was neurotic. Only four years after her symptoms began did she have a full assessment and brain scan and was given a definite diagnosis of Alzheimer dementia. The uncertainly was over; her family were devastated, but she was relieved.

Her struggle to get a definite diagnosis is typical. Research by the Alzheimer's Society indicates that a shocking 60% of those with dementia in UK never receive a diagnosis. Many doctors fail to diagnose the condition early because they rely too much on tests of remembering facts.

Jennifer resigned and retired, but amazingly she saw her fearful diagnosis as a chance to help others and even called it a "glorious opportunity". After starting medication, her ability to communicate improved. With the help of family and friends she set up a wonderful website, gave interviews and prepared leaflets to educate those with dementia, their carers and the health professions. Her experience of how she used the early years of her Alzheimer's disease are very positive. Even though her condition has progressed and she is now in a special village for those with dementia, she is still doing valuable advisory work after about 20 years!

Her story is remarkable. She moved from apparent calamity to the opportunity to share and care.

Read more about her and what she is still doing on her website: *www.gloriousopportunity.org.*

Frank and Linda

DEMENTIA: FRANK AND LINDA'S STORY[21]

> *With dementia life changes, but there are strategies to help, cope and care. There can still be years of meaningful life.*

This story and the valuable advice that goes with it are modified from *Dementia: Frank and Linda's Story* by Louise Morse and published by Monarch Books (2010).

[21] Louise Morse; *Dementia: Frank and Linda's Story;* Monarch Books (2010).

Frank has dementia. Now he is 72, but it had been diagnosed when he was 66. Linda had suspected there was something wrong before that because sometimes he could not find the right word, he lost things and repeated himself. He had been a good driver, but this had changed, little by little; he tended to stay near the line in the middle of the road and sometimes lost his way to places he knew. He even drove into their neighbour's driveway by mistake, had a minor accident and reluctantly accepted that he would have to give up driving! He was more anxious and sometimes depressed; this could have been because there were redundancies at work and he had to retire early, but also he could not do what he used to do. Frustrating!

Linda was now 70 and had been good at multitasking as she had needed to bring up a family, but was now slowed down by arthritis. She realised that Frank was changing and she had to adapt and adopt strategies to cope. Frank had always been easygoing, but now he was easily irritated. Even simple things could be complicated, for example helping Frank to put on his socks. Sometimes he would object because he thought that they were not his or they did not feel right. After giving up driving, he sometimes tried to get into the driver's seat and Linda would say, "Please sit next to me; that gives me the confidence I need when I have to drive." At home, she learnt how to distract him with his favourite DVD of the 'Dam Busters' and a cup of tea.

Frank had always helped Linda with the housework, but with dementia his help took on an extra dimension. When Linda was busy in the kitchen, about twice a week, Frank would rearrange the furniture in the lounge but would forget he had done it and could not explain why. He would tidy things away, and quite often put useful items into the rubbish bin in the kitchen. If she asked him where the keys or the clothes brush had gone he would look worried, even alarmed. She needed a range of strategies to cope with these activities; for example, she used to keep clean liners in the bin so she could search for things. When Frank was headed towards the rubbish bin with a vase of flowers, Linda intercepted: "Thank you, Frank, how clever of you to notice that the vase needed to be topped up." It was a constant and stressful job!

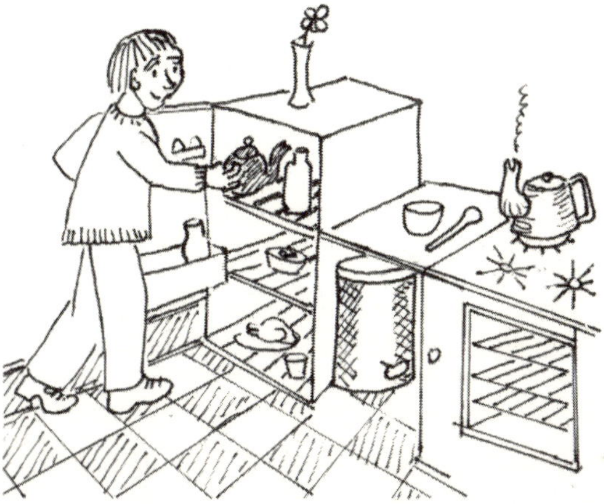

A life of surprises. The tea pot in the fridge.

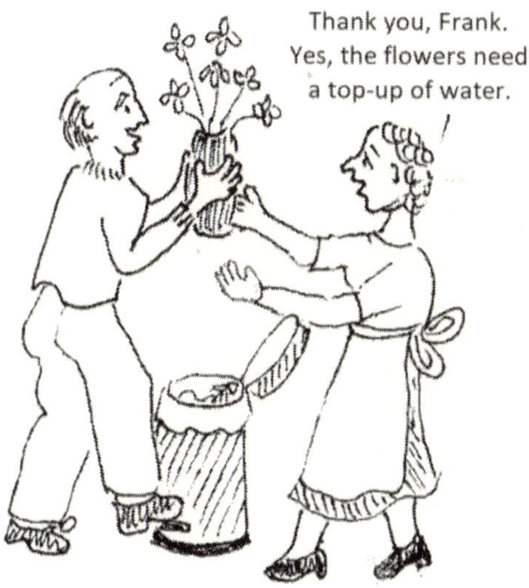
Thank you, Frank.
Yes, the flowers need
a top-up of water.

Flowers rescued!

For Linda, life before dementia (BD) and after dementia (AD) were very different. BD life was straightforward and predictable; things would move in the usual manner. But AD, life was complicated, tense and sometimes Frank did unexpected things. Linda had to use different strategies to keep him from doing things that could cause harm, like locking doors to stop him walking out of the house and getting lost. In a later chapter, the range of more disturbing symptoms and signs of dementia will be briefly reviewed, with suggestions about ways to cope with the many challenges.

Obviously, dementia affects every aspect of life: physical, mental, social and even spiritual. Frank and Linda had to adjust in all these spheres.

Could it be dementia?

WHY DIAGNOSIS IS OFTEN DIFFICULT AND SLOW

Over half the people with the condition in Britain in 2014 were not given the diagnosis. For both Frank and Jennifer Bute, it took years while they struggled not knowing what was happening to themselves. When it was confirmed, despite its ominous implications, they felt some sense of relief.

First, there is an overlap between a natural slowing of bodily functions with age and the early symptoms of dementia. Most Seniors may find it difficult to remember the names of people and places, this is called Mild Cognitive Impairment (MCI) which is not dementia. But this could be a sign of the start of dementia.

There are also problems with doctors and the health service. Many General Practitioners (family doctors) have not had recent training about dementia. The simple test that they apply mainly checks recall (short-term memory) and not reasoning or wider brain functions.

Also, doctors may be reluctant to 'label' a patient with such a serious diagnosis because of the stigma and the life-limiting implications of this disease.

It is not known why the course of disease is more rapid in some people than others or why some brains are functionally resilient despite showing signs of dementia on examination.[22] It is possible that some 'rewiring' to bypass blocked brain circuits is possible. This happens in a few patients after brain damage from a stroke. Perhaps these people have adopted activities that have limited disease progression. No wonder some doctors hesitate about labelling a person with this diagnosis.

WHAT SHOULD YOU DO IF YOU ARE WORRIED?

Are you concerned that either you or a relative has dementia? Neither panic nor denial is sensible. The diagnosis of dementia is a process; it is not a simple one-off like a blood test. After all, there are many conditions that cause dementia, even though about 60% have Alzheimer's disease. If you have real doubts, do not evade the process. An early diagnosis can be useful because there are many useful things that can be done.

- First, check the symptoms from the common symptoms list on page 53.
- Consult your General Practitioner (family doctor) who will probably give you a general check up to make sure any slow-down is not caused by some other condition like poor thyroid function. He or she may give you a mini-memory test and request an X-ray or scan of your brain.
- Your GP may then refer you to a memory clinic or to a neurologist or psychologist.
- The specialist may order more detailed tests and a brain scan. This is usually an MRI (Magnetic Resonance Imaging), which does not involve X-rays but gives clear pictures of the size and structure of the brain.

After all of that, the specialists should be able to give you a reliable answer. Even if the answer is that you do have dementia, there are many useful things that you can do. Take courage; be positive with the prospect of years of enjoyable life.

---

[22] See the nuns study on page 50.

In Lighter Mode: Puns

Laugh-age is essential on the journey of life,
even when it punishes the English langu-age.

The pun, also called paronomasia, is a form of humorous wordplay that exploits the multiple meanings of words, or of similar-sounding words. Apologies for a few medical puns and other simple jokes!

Seniors are like puns; they are the simplest form of wit.

I had decided against a brain transplant, but then I changed my mind.

I heard this joke about amnesia, but I forget how it goes.

Claustrophobic people are more productive thinking outside the box.

A sign on the lawn at a drug rehab centre said, "Keep off the grass."

The letter from the clinic said I had type-A blood, but it was a type-O.

A little boy swallowed some small coins and was taken to a hospital. When his grandmother telephoned to ask how he was, a nurse said, "No change yet."

The surgeon told the patient, "I'll have to remove the whole left side, then you will be all right."

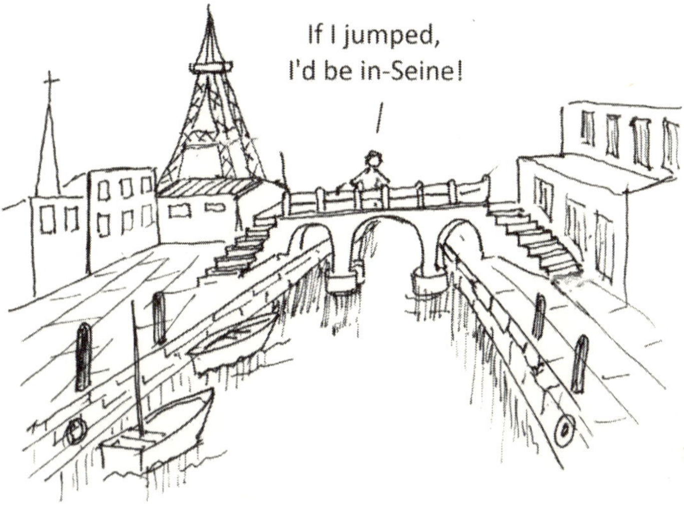

Crazy suicide attempt in Paris.

Jill broke her finger today, but on the other hand she was completely fine.

Did you hear about the Buddhist who refused local anaesthetic during drilling a root canal? His goal: transcend dental medication.

The soldier who survived mustard gas and pepper spray is now a seasoned veteran.

At the football match the man was hit on the head with a can of soda. It could have been serious, but luckily it was a soft drink.

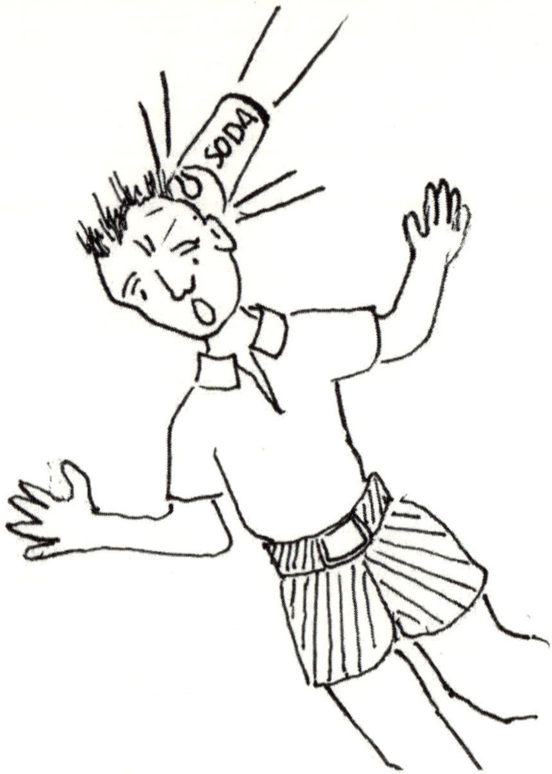

Soda strike.

CHAPTER THREE

What is Going On? Understanding Dementia

Memory is so important to every person. It enables us to learn, retain and recall information. Because of our memory we modify our behaviour in the light of earlier experience and we function as individuals. Memory gives us our sense of who we are; our identity. Without it we are frightened and lost.

What is dementia? A brief summary

Dementia is a general name for conditions that gradually damage many functions of the brain: at first, remembering, thinking and reasoning, and later many other functions like moving, talking and eating. The term "decline in cognitive function" is often used. This simply means the person is now "less able to think, remember, work things out and communicate".

Alzheimer's disease is the most common form of dementia, accounting for about 60% of all diagnosed cases in older people.

LOSS OF MEMORY AND COGNITIVE FUNCTION, THINKING AND COMMUNICATING

As the human body gets older it is normal for the organs and tissues to show signs of age and they do not function so well. We sometimes say, "It's just wear and tear." It is normal for older

Seniors to slow down and become forgetful of some things, for example remembering the names of people, even people they know quite well. However, there is a significant difference between forgetting where you put your car keys and forgetting what the car keys are used for, forgetting where you left your coat and remembering how to put it on. The first can be called normal elderly forgetfulness, but the second would be considered a sign of dementia.

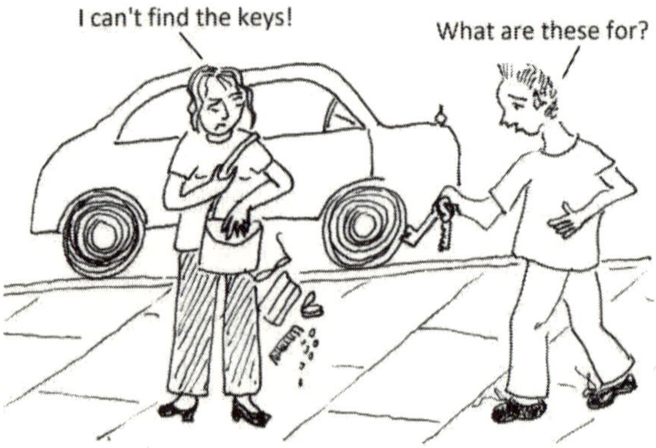

The car keys.

The brain stores different sorts of information in different ways, and sometimes in different parts of the brain.

One classification of memory is between recent, short-term facts and information and long-term memory from years ago, even from childhood. Often those with dementia have poor short-term memory but relatively well preserved long-term memory.

Another classification of memory is between explicit and implicit memory. Explicit memory is the recall of facts and events, especially things you learnt or were involved in recently. The term 'episodic' memory is sometimes used for forgetfulness of what has just happened recently.

Implicit memory has different components: skills and habits you learnt and repeated like riding a cycle or knitting, also musical memory, tunes, songs and hymns that have particular associations. It includes emotional associations with certain smells and fragrances, or situations associated with joy and fear, comfort and security. Because of this, people with quite advanced disease can appreciate and remember friendship, kindness and caresses, even if they cannot express their appreciation. There is evidence that implicit memory is stored in different and specific parts of the brain.

In Alzheimer's disease, explicit memory (recently learnt facts) appears to fail while implicit memory (musical, habitual and emotional memory) lasts longer. Rejoice for nostalgia! – long-term and emotional memory are better preserved than memory of recent trivia!

Factors known to have some role in dementia include age, lifestyle, environment and genetic inheritance. This last, the genetic inheritance, has only about a quarter of the power of the other factors.[23]

Uncertainty about the nature of the disease process

The causes of brain failure – mechanical, blocked nerve pathways or biochemical, neuro-transmission breakdown – are still not fully understood. This is admitted in the latest book on the subject, Joseph Jebelli's *In Pursuit of Memory*[24]. In dementia, the death and loss of many neurones (brain cells) causes brain shrinkage in specific areas, but the cause of cell death is not certain.

In the brains of many patients with Alzheimer's disease are tangles of a protein called tau and plaques of amyloid material believed to inhibit normal brain cell function. Major drug trials of anti-amyloid drugs have been shown to reduce brain amyloid

---

[23] See chapter 11 on prevention.

[24] J. Jebelli; *In pursuit of memory. The fight against Alzheimer's;* Hodder and Stoughton (2017).

without improving cognition, brain function.[25] This means that current understanding of the disease mechanism is still very incomplete with no 'cure' in sight.

Following the failure of anti-amyloid treatments to improve brain function, attention is turning away from amyloid to inflammation, allergy or autoimmune degeneration affecting microglial cells of the brain. These are resident immune cells that constitute about 10-15% of brain cells and they sustain normal neurotransmission between neurones. One hypothesis is that damaged or activated microglial cells impair nerve transmissions or kill neurones.

DIFFERENCES BRAIN STRUCTURE AND BRAIN FUNCTION

In some careful studies, the clinical features, the cognitive function and the performance of individuals did not match fully with the anatomical appearance and pathological findings in their brains.

A long-term study of 700 retired nuns, many of them former teachers, was started in Minnesota, USA in 1986.[26] They were given a range of physical and mental tests over fifteen years and a number developed the clinical features of Alzheimer's disease. All these nuns had consented to leave their brains for pathological examination after they died and these were all removed, examined and analysed. There was poor correlation between the neuropathology features of Alzheimer's in the brain and poor cognitive function during life. In some who had significant Alzheimer's, pathology of their brains were resilient, retaining cognition, memory and comprehension. On the contrary, some who had clinical features of dementia had brains that appeared normal in appearance on examination.

---

[25] LeCouteur D.G., Hunter S., Brayne C.; *Solanezumab and the amyloid hypothesis for Alzheimer's disease;* BMJ (29 Dec 2016); 355 *https://doi.org/10.1136/bmj.i6771;* BMJ 2016;355:i6771.

[26] Negash S., et al.; *Resilient brain aging: characterization of discordance between Alzheimer's disease pathology and cognition;* Curr Alzheimer Res. (Oct 2013);10(8):844-51; *www.ncbi.nlm.nihgov/pubmed/23919768*

This interesting and puzzling study simply emphasizes our limited understanding of the basic causes of dementia and the features seen in the brains of those with Alzheimer's disease.

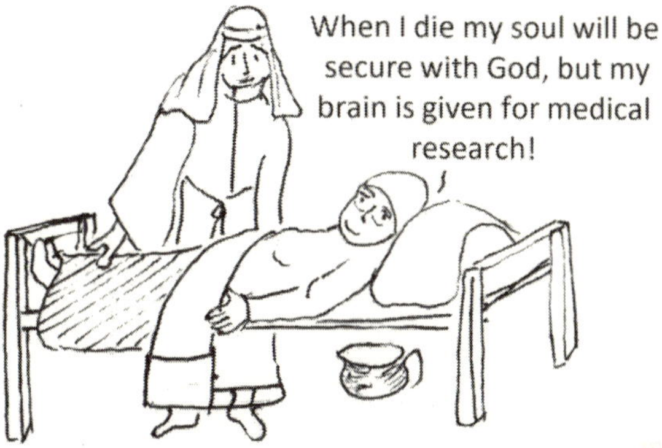

The dying nun's donation.

Types of dementia

There are a number of types of dementia:

- *Alzheimer's disease* often develops slowly over several years, is not always obvious to begin with and symptoms can be subtle and overlap with other illnesses such as depression. This is the commonest type.
- *Vascular dementia* is the second commonest type, caused by poor or blocked blood supply to parts of the brain. This may be associated with patients who have damage to the heart and blood vessels. Some people have both vascular dementia and Alzheimer's disease – often called *mixed dementia.*
- *Dementia with Lewy bodies* (DLB) has slightly different features, sometimes with movement problems like Parkinson's disease.
- *Fronto-temporal dementia,* so called because it mainly affects those parts of the brain, may cause sufferers to have

more behaviour problems like agitation and aggression and sometimes language difficulties.

- *Post-traumatic dementia:* it is now recognised that accident head injuries and a number of sports injuries can be associated with dementia.

Progress of dementia

As different areas of the brain stop working properly, there are different effects: symptoms and signs, memory loss, mood changes and problems with reasoning, communicating with others, carrying out daily activities and abnormal behaviour. Ultimately, because the brain controls all body functions, the person can no longer move, communicate or swallow and becomes completely dependent on care. All forms of dementia slowly deteriorate to a helpless state where patients need help with nearly everything and ultimately respiration and circulation fail. A number of those with dementia die from cancer or heart and blood vessel diseases before they die from dementia.

The rate of deterioration varies, more quickly in some people and more slowly in others, from two or three years to more than ten or twenty. There can be years of contented life and even useful work as Dr Jennifer Bute demonstrates.

Some people who have been diagnosed and labelled as having dementia seem to manage a simple lifestyle for years if they are well supported by family and friends.

STAGES

The condition is simply divided into *early* stage (mild), *medium* stage (moderate) and *late* stage (severe) according to how dependent the patient is on personal care.

Symptoms and signs

Dementia is recognised from a set of symptoms when the brain is damaged by the conditions described above.

The symptom list below is from the comprehensive Alzheimer's Association website[27] and also from Dr Jennifer Bute's writings and website[28].

COMMON SYMPTOMS IN EARLY STAGE DEMENTIA

The story of Frank and Linda showed that Frank had many common signs and symptoms of dementia, and some features of more progressive disease. Below is a more comprehensive list.

These are more than the normal changes of getting old:

- Increasing memory loss. It's not just forgetting where you put something, but how to use it.
- People with dementia sometimes have depression. However, depression can be an illness on its own and not a part of dementia.
- Inability to work things out and understanding the significance of events.
- Not finding the right word or names for things. Forgetting people's names is common. Forgetting how they relate to your life is more significant.
- Losing your way, sometimes even in places you know.
- Misplacing items, putting them away in the wrong places.
- Loss of confidence and anxiety about failing to remember.
- Difficulty making decisions and difficulty learning new things.
- Losing interest in things you used to enjoy.

LIVING IN AN EARLIER WORLD IN MEDIUM STAGE DEMENTIA

People with dementia often have a very different perception of the world. Short-term memory goes and so they may not know where they are or whom they are with. Penny Garner and Oliver

---

27 *www.alzheimers.org.uk*

28 *www.gloriousopportunity.org*

James describe memory as a big photograph album.[29] There are lots of pictures from long ago that are well fixed onto the pages, but some of the recent pictures (memories) have not been well fixed and are missing from the pages. Some people with dementia live in "a past memory world" that is more real to them than what they have recently heard or seen. Some old folk re-enact something from their earlier life. If you tell them that their picture of present reality is wrong, they become upset and anxious.

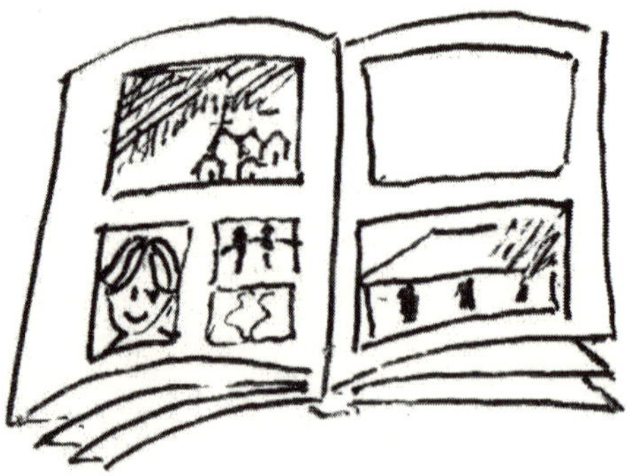

The memory photo album, with pictures missing.

SYMPTOMS WHEN THE DISEASE PROGRESSES, IN MEDIUM AND LATE STAGE

Not everyone will have all or the same set of symptoms.

- Repeating questions.
- Tiredness, lethargy and sleeping more than usual.
- Getting out of the normal routine and not realising it.
- Difficulty with simple tasks like choosing clothes and getting meals.
- Not wanting to get dressed and go out of the home.

[29] Oliver James; *Contented Dementia;* Vermilion, Ebony Publishing (2008). (Also see chapter entitled 'Comfortable Dementia – The SPECAL Method of Care' on page 151.)

- Not taking care of the home when this had been seen as important.
- Misjudging things, like wearing the wrong clothes for the weather and not recognising danger.
- Personal hygiene deteriorates, clothes stained and hair not tidied.
- Losing interest in family, friends and hobbies.
- Forgetting the normal rules of courtesy and social skills.
- Rapid changes of mood for no obvious reason.
- Personality changes; becoming apathetic, confused or suspicious.
- Withdrawing from social contact and deepening depression.
- Increasing difficulty with reading or writing.
- If some parts of the brain are affected: hallucinations, seeing things that are not there and delusions experiencing non-existing smells or sounds.
- Difficulty in swallowing food.
- Incontinence.
- Inability to comprehend, talk and communicate.

Clearly these last three signs have major social and practical consequences.

BEHAVIOUR MAY CHANGE

Because the brain controls how we interact with the world and other people, if parts of the brain do not work, behaviour may change and this can be disturbing. This is not a mental illness. The behaviour may be simple, like repeating questions or repeating actions like dusting, or agitation which may mean that the person is anxious or in discomfort. Other issues are walking about (wandering), inside or outside the home, abusive language, reluctance to eat or bath and inappropriate sexual behaviour.

If the part of the brain that effects emotions is damaged or uncontrolled, then a person may speak or act in an uninhibited or shocking manner, as they have never done before. They do not set out to be awkward or behave badly.

Sometimes the behaviour indicates that the person does not understand what is going on, or is trying to communicate something and struggles to get the message across. This may be because of:

- Physical discomfort, needing the toilet, illness, or medication side effects.
- Overstimulation, such as loud noise or an environment that is too busy.
- Unfamiliar surroundings, such as a new place or inability to recognise an old one.
- Too complicated a task or difficulty with tasks or activities.
- Frustrating interactions, such as inability to communicate effectively.

For carers, many of whom are close relatives, these changes and behaviour are difficult to deal with, emotionally stressful and they wear you down. Remember that the behaviour is the result of the disease; it is not deliberately hurtful. Try to respond calmly and do not hesitate to ask for help from others. See the many practical points in chapter 8 on care and coping with dementia.

In Lighter Mode: Two Figures

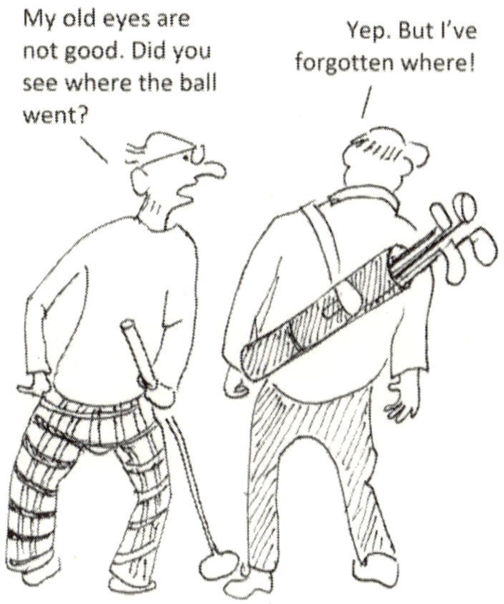
My old eyes are not good. Did you see where the ball went?
Yep. But I've forgotten where!

Old golfers' limitations.

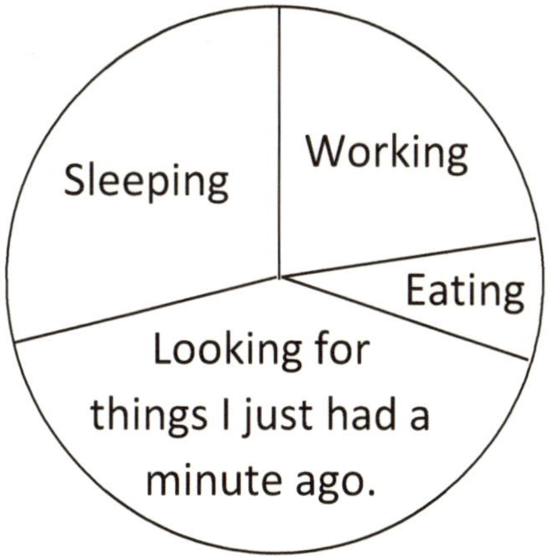
Sleeping
Working
Eating
Looking for things I just had a minute ago.

How Seniors spend their time.

In Lighter Mode: Older and Wiser

Is slow response due to information overload, not to memory decline?
Dr. Michael Ramscar of the University of Tuebingen in Germany, concluded, "The performance of older adults reflects increased knowledge, not cognitive decline."
You can kid your friends about this, say, "The grey-matter disc is full; plenty of information there, only retrieval is slow."
But most neurologists don't agree with him.

Chapter Four

Spiritual Strength for the Dementia Journey

Dementia and Alzheimer's disease: these words cause alarm and distress in the hearts and minds of most people.

Much of this book describes the physical, mental and social consequences of the condition and how best to live with and combat the effects of this disease. As already mentioned, the emotional and music memories often last and linger along with the capacity to feel deeply, emotionally and spiritually.

Christians believe that God is important to every sphere of life. Many Christians have found that having a spiritual dimension can give strength, direction and assurance for every stage of life. This certainly includes periods of illness and dementia. In this chapter are some of the experiences that have been helpful on the dementia journey.

LOOK BACK AT FRANK AND LINDA'S STORY

Frank said, "Getting the diagnosis – dementia – was a shock, but also a sense of relief. What's been happening to me is a physical illness in my brain. I'm not going mad!"

He and Linda were practising Christians and they set about dealing with things in a positive way. The Bible tells us that believers will have to go through trials of all sorts. We are pilgrims, on our way to "a new heaven and a new earth"[30] where we know that things will be better. Better than we can imagine.

Meanwhile, we have to live positively on this earth with its pile of problems! The Bible has a lot of encouragement for people going through difficult times, times of feeling helpless, frightened and lonely.

Foundational beliefs

For Christians, any understanding of dementia must be built on theological and biblical foundations.

First is the recognition that our God is a powerful creator, a gracious sustainer and a loving redeemer of men and women. Any meaning for our individual lives does not depend on our actions or achievements, or on our thoughts or our memories. Only by God's thought and love were we created and are we sustained. Only by his intervention through Jesus Christ can we be redeemed. Our only eternal significance and identity is that God continues to keep us in his thoughts and love!

Second, the Bible tells us that God's nature is one of love and concern for the vulnerable and helpless. Those affected by dementia or Alzheimer's disease certainly fit that category.

Third, Christian believers are gathered in a community of faith, the church, which is sustained by God's Holy Spirit and is active in the world. It is a community in which help and hope are found.

In the next three sections we see three aspects of God's nature that are relevant to people living with dementia:

1. GOD HAS A SPECIAL LOVE FOR THE HELPLESS

The Bible tells us that God's nature is one of love and concern for the helpless. Throughout its pages we learn that He has a deep compassion for those who are unable to protect themselves and may be vulnerable and open to abuse. This theme shines out from

[30] Revelation 21:1.

every part of the Bible, from the initial statements about the nature of God in Genesis, through the songs of psalmists and the pronouncements of the prophets, to the words and the deeds of Jesus. Jesus teaches and demonstrates that God is committed to people in need, having a heart for the vulnerable – and this definitely includes those with dementia.

The Old Testament declares:

> *He defends the cause of the fatherless and the widow, and loves the foreigner residing among you, giving them food and clothing.*
>
> *Deuteronomy 10:18 (NIV)*

> *You listen to the longings of those who suffer. You offer them hope, and you pay attention to their cries for help.*
>
> *Psalm 10:17 (CEV)*

Sadly, the selfish and violent actions of men have often opposed and apparently frustrated the intentions of God.

In the New Testament the same theme of concerned love is repeated despite the persecution of God's people.

> *When we were utterly helpless, Christ came at just the right time and died for us sinners.*
>
> *Romans 5:6 (NLT)*

> *No, I will not abandon you as orphans – I will come to you.*
>
> *John 14:18 (NLT)*

Paul reminds the Christians in Corinth that...

> *God deliberately chose men and women that the culture overlooks and exploits and abuses, he chose these "nobodies" to expose the hollow pretensions of the "celebrities".*
>
> *1 Corinthians 1:27 (MSG)*

These verses are a few of many speaking of God's concern for the vulnerable. Printed as a list they may seem out of context, but the theme is certainly present. God loves those who are helpless, lost, lonely, isolated or in trouble, and that surely describes those with advanced dementia.

Jesus had a special compassion for those who were paralysed, epileptic or outcast because of their abnormal behaviour. We know this from the stories of his interaction and healing love for such people. We can be sure that...

> *God has a special love for just such people as those with dementia.*

2. GOD'S CHILDREN ARE CONSTANTLY IN THE THOUGHTS OF A LOVING FATHER

The fact that God created, sustains and redeemed human life indicates that he cares for and loves men and women. He made man with intellect and memory, and capable of love and other responses and relationships.

From many parts of the Bible we recognise that God declares that people should be cared for. This includes even those who do not have a fully functional body or brain. A newborn baby has no intellectual capacity and no memory, but is already in relationship to a family and of course is worthy of love and care. Likewise, a person with dementia may have limited intellectual reasoning and incomplete memory, but is still a member of the human family and worthy of love and care. Of even greater significance, every person is in the heart and mind of God, one of his loved children and worthy of love and care. A person may have forgotten who he or she is, but each person is still in the heart and memory of God. And that is most important.

Review and remember the key story that Jesus told, 'The Prodigal Son'. [31] Justifiably, it could have been called 'The Parable

---

[31] Luke 15:11-24.

of the Loving Father'. The young man in the far country was taken up first with prostitutes and then with pigs. But all the while, the father was thinking of and looking out for his son. God always holds his children in his heart and mind. Even if I have forgotten who I am, my most profound existence, my most significant identity, is that I am in the thoughts and memory of my loving Father God. This core message is of fundamental importance.

3. GOD WATCHES OVER HIS CHILDREN

We know that we are God's greatly loved children, and those living with dementia are still God's children!

> *See how very much our Father loves us, for he calls us his children, and that is what we are!*
>
> *1 John 3:1 (GNB)*

In every part of the Bible we read that God does not abandon us. Like the prodigal's father, his eyes are constantly on the look-out for his child.

Psalm 139 tells us that we are continuously in the sight and the mind of our Lord God. Again it tells us that God seeks and watches over his children. In verses 7-12 it emphasizes that no geographic distance, no darkness as deep as death is beyond God's vision. He sees and protects his own.

> *Where could I go to escape from your Spirit or from your sight?*
> *If I were to climb up to the highest heavens, you would be there.*
> *If I were to dig down to the world of the dead you would also be there.*
> *Suppose I had wings like the dawning day and flew across the ocean.*
> *Even then your powerful arm would guide and protect me.*

Or suppose I said, "I'll hide in the dark until night comes to cover me over." But you see in the dark because daylight and dark are all the same to you.

Psalm 139:7-12 (CEV)

To those who trust in God he has ultimately promised in heaven a new body, and surely that will include a new brain. It will have a structure and function beyond our speculation.[32]

Remembering and rementing

DAVID'S STORY

Pastor David Roper wrote about his friend's husband who was in the last stages of dementia. He was admitted to a care home and when first introduced to the nurse who was to care for him, he reached out for her arm and stopped her. He said, "May I introduce you to my best friend? He loves me deeply."

Since no one else was in the room, the nurse thought he was hallucinating. But for a few minutes he spoke clearly about Jesus and what he meant to him. She was deeply touched, but had to move on to the next room to care for another patient. When she returned, the darkness had closed in again and the man was mute and no longer lucid.

Even though this man had descended into the darkest phase of dementia, he knew that the Lord was his best friend. God can reach down to the greatest depths to which a soul can fall. His light can penetrate the deepest darkness and assure us of his tender loving care. Indeed no darkness will hide us from him. Even in the depth of dementia the Lord's hand will hold us, his powerful arm will guide and protect us! We cannot get away from his love and personal care. That is the promise in Psalm 139.

> *Christian faith can be a strength on the journey.*

[32] 2 Corinthians 5:1.

REMEMBERING

When people get old, even if they do not have dementia, they may appear frail, fragile and pathetic. Even those close to them may not realise, or may forget, that in their time they were leaders, trendsetters, role models; courageous, hard-working; dynamic mothers; holding together families, communities, companies and even countries.

When my friend, Dr Peter Little, saw his parents getting old and frail, he remembered all the good and great things that they had done. He wanted to honour them with gratitude and he wrote a short poem for them.

> You are not WHAT you are
> But WHO you are
> And you still own
> Everything you have ever been and done.

When dementia or Alzheimer's disease robs a person of memory, cognition and communication, it is easy to forget the real person they were. Even their nearest and dearest may forget what they really were.

Christians firmly believe that even if much of the brain has been destroyed, the soul remains. The real person is still there, fully remembered, known to and deeply loved by God, and worthy of care and respect.

The theologian Dr John Swinton[33] declared that...

> *Our memories do not make us what we are;*
> *we are what God remembers us to be.*
> *One of his children and precious in his sight.*[34]

[33] Rev. Dr. Joanna Collicutt; *Thinking of you;* Bible Reading Fellowship (Abingdon, 2017). In this section I am grateful for the work and inspiration of Dr Collicutt.

[34] John Swinton in: Sally Magnuson; *Where Memories Go – Why dementia changes everything;* Two Roads (2014); page 328.

REMENTING

David's story, above, is one of *rementing*. This is a word used to mean a lucid moment, a brief remission from memory and cognitive absence, when someone mute with dementia speaks or sings. Sometimes it is evoked by music, a scent or a conversation. Occasionally, it may be associated with a special spiritual vision or a message and is believed to be a brief visitation of the Holy Spirit.

Dr Jennifer Bute tells a story about her father who had been a committed Christian but he developed severe Alzheimer's and had not spoken for months. After watching Songs of Praise on the TV, the leader said a prayer and concluded with, "Amen," and Jennifer's dad joined in with a loud amen of his own.

She asked him, "Dad, do you still pray?" Then, after an affirmative grunt, she asked him, "What do you say to God?"

After a pregnant pause, he replied, "Hello."

Wonderful! A comfortable greeting between friends!

There are times, even in advanced dementia, when 'the fog rolls back' and you can see the person as they were. This rementing happens sometimes when in a meeting, singing familiar songs or hymns, or during a time of prayer; a person who has not spoken for ages will respond with an appropriate comment or prayer. These are real but fleeting times of insight when you glimpse the real person is still there.

David's story, given above, is another example of such a rementing.

Friendship and fellowship during the dementia journey

There is no doubt that care from a personal friend or a spouse is one of the greatest comforts and benefits during this journey. Those who live in relative isolation may go downhill much more rapidly. An old couple may both have memories that frequently fail, but they can complement each other and trigger a larger range of memories and even jokes!

THE COMPANIONSHIP OF CHRIST ON THE DEMENTIA JOURNEY

Two Christian ladies who have dementia have lived remarkable and productive lives for many years after diagnosis. They are both stalwart campaigners for positive life with dementia.

Jennifer Bute[35] was asked, "What difference has it made to your life with dementia that you have a Christian faith?"

"Everything!" she replied. "Nothing is wasted in God's economy. I see my dementia as an unexpected gift from God. Like pain, it's not comfortable, but I believe it is a great privilege for me to understand it from the inside. It has enriched my life. I ask God to help me rejoice in adversity. Others see my joy. Now, living in a dementia-friendly village, I am able to walk this path with many others and encourage them to find God's love."[36]

Christine Bryden was an Australian Government Executive in her forties when diagnosed with dementia. After over twenty years from diagnosis, she is still positive about the disease and a passionate campaigner against the stigma of the condition and for a dementia-friendly society.

Like Dr Jennifer Bute, her Christian faith is an important factor in her life and approach to the condition. In her book, *Dancing with Dementia: My story of living positively with dementia,* she says:

> *For me, healing is wholeness of the body, mind and spirit … I know that I have been healed spiritually of the doubt of where God might be in all of this, and of the fear of the disease itself, the way that it takes away the mind bit by bit. This spiritual and emotional healing happened in stages for me. I am living the experience of a more holistic healing. I can also say that I am not*

---

[35] See page 37.

[36] Jennifer Bute; *The Gift of Years. Bible reflections for older people. January-April 2017;* Bible Reading Fellowship (Abingdon, 2017).

declining with dementia as fast as expected. ... I know that spiritual healing is the greater eternal solution. All of this is God's work and my neurologist in Sydney never ceases to be amazed at my level of functioning despite steady brain deterioration.[37]

She declares:

Its a terrible diagnosis to have, but think positively. I really believe there's a new life to be lived in the slow lane of dementia.

A DEMENTIA-FRIENDLY CHURCH AND COMMUNITY

The concern of God for the vulnerable and stranger calls his Church to be a caring community within the larger community. With the recognition that there are many with dementia in all societies, the Christian Church should be at the forefront of befriending and accommodating those with the condition and their carers.[38]

The Church and its individual members must demonstrate Jesus' love, care and companionship to those whose lives appear to be falling apart. It should be willing to identify with these people with empathy, authenticity and affection, so this is no quick, easy or casual relationship. Sometimes it means travelling with people in their irrational worries into 'the land of forgetfulness' and occasionally into "the valley of the shadow of death"[39].

There are some solid practicalities for a dementia-friendly church (DFC) to start with. The access should be easy, preferably

[37] Christine Bryden; *Dancing with Dementia. My story of living positively with dementia;* Jessica Kingsley Publishers (2005).

[38] Rosie Barker; *Six Key Steps to Making a DEMENTIA FRIENDLY Church;* Pilgrims' Friend Society (London); *info@pilgrimsfriend.org.uk.*
Revd Dr Margaret Goodall and Gaynor Hammond; *Growing Dementia Friendly Churches. A Practical Guide;* Christians on Ageing (North Allerton); *info@ccoa.org.uk.*

[39] Psalm 23:4 (KJV).

with a ramp. Inside, the lighting should be good, the labelling clear, colours strong, the atmosphere warm, toilets accessible and preferably a loop system to help those with hearing aids.

The human touch is even more important: a warm welcome at the door and friendship after worship. To achieve this, the leadership should be fully committed to the vision of a DFC without compromising other important sections of the congregation. Project leaders in the wider congregation should model love, sensitivity and some flexibility so those with dementia can worship in a simple manner.

Hopefully, some members of the congregation will learn some of the simple guidelines about communicating with those who have dementia. These include: approach from the front, make eye contact, do not start by asking them questions, don't contradict or interrupt, and bear with repetition. It is good to have a 'buddy', a special church friend for each person with dementia, someone who will help, explain what is going on and will be a regular contact in the church.

BARBARA'S STORY

Barbara was very forgetful and needed much help to be sure she looked after herself safely. Each Sunday, Betty called to take her to church.

"Sometimes I forget who I am, but when I'm in church with Betty, I hear the Bible stories and sing the familiar hymns. Then I know I'm safe in God's love."

A DFC needs to keep in touch with its own members who develop the condition and visit them regularly, listen with empathy and find out what is important for them. Always affirm that the person is still a valued child of God. Some churches have memory clubs or host small events to stimulate memories. Some have simplified forms of worship in which those with more advanced condition can participate. The person may only be able to engage a little but it is important that they are given the opportunity. Some with dementia and a deep faith may worry about how they can remember God. To say to them that God remembers them may be enough, but it is important to support their personal life of prayer and Bible study for as long as possible.

MABEL'S STORY

Mabel was a widow and knew that her memory was getting unreliable. She started to feel embarrassed about going out in case she did something stupid. She was getting more isolated. Her friend Laura asked her, "Would you like to come with me to church next Sunday? There is a friendly group of people there." Laura met and took her, sat with her and explained what was going on in the service.

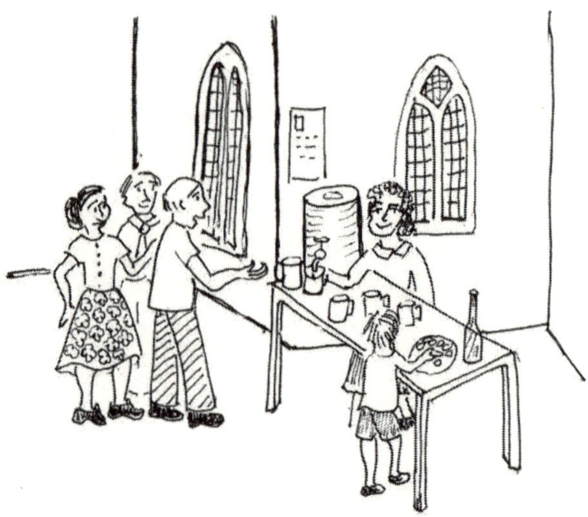

Mabel said, "I feel comfortable and useful helping to serve coffee."

Mabel went a couple more times and then said to Laura, "I had not been to church for many years, but I feel comfortable there with your friends. I remember the amazing Bible stories, enjoy the old hymns and even some of the new lively ones. I feel welcome and at home."

Before long she had made a few new friends and started to help to make the coffee! She felt she belonged and she began to believe and put her trust in Jesus and his promises for her future. She went from belonging to believing – and to a deeper life.

AUDREY'S STORY

Sitting in the church hall having coffee after the service, a group of older folk were laughing and sharing stories. Audrey said, "I love it here; I don't feel like I have dementia when I come here."

One of her friends responded, "We forget about your dementia when you're here."

Audrey answered, "Well I forget everything else; I might as well forget about my dementia!"

Everyone saw the funny side of her joke and laughed with her.

Fun and laughter are invaluable weapons against ever-lurking anxieties. This is success; everyone forgot about the dementia and focused on the person. God's Spirit was in the love and friendship of that group!

In the Gospel of Matthew, Jesus said that what we do for the least of his brothers and sisters we do for him.

> *For I was hungry and you fed me; I was thirsty and you gave me water; I was a stranger and you invited me into your homes; naked and you clothed me; sick and in prison and you visited me.*
>
> *Matthew 25:35-45*

Today, Jesus, with a group of people, might say, "I was hungry for understanding and thirsty for friendship and you visited me. I was a stranger in the strange land of dementia, lost, lonely and vulnerable and you visited me. I was in the prison of my confused and blank mind, but you visited me and your kindness and love made me feel like a free person again."

Spiritual supports during the dementia journey

The Book of Proverbs (4:23) states:

Above everything else, guard your heart;
for it is the source of life's consequences…

Proverbs 4:23 (CJB)

But how can we 'guard our hearts'?
Here are some practical suggestions:

- Prayers.
- Meditation and mindfulness.
- Rituals and reminders.

PRAYERS

People living with dementia may be encouraged to pray. Spiritual life can continue!

One good thing about prayer is that it can be simple. It does not require intellectual training or erudite words, but it is opening your heart to God in wonder, gratitude, love or desperation.

But some discipline is good. God is ready for our urgent prayers when we feel anxious, but his 'line' is open for any-time prayers, whenever you simply need to chat.

Encourage all Seniors, including those with dementia, to set aside a regular time for devotions and prayer each day. 'The quiet time', a period set aside every day for Bible reading and prayer, has been used and valued by many over years and centuries.

If friends with early dementia are up to reading, there are now specific daily Bible reading notes for Seniors, for example:

- *Prayers for Seniors*[40] by William Barclay is a booklet of simple prayers for morning and evening with additional prayers for the situations of older people.

---

[40] William Barclay; *Prayers for Seniors;* St Paul's Press (Mumbai, India). Copies also available from Dr W. A. M. Cutting, 80 Abingdon Road, Cumnor, Oxon. OX2 9QW, UK.

- *50 Services of Christian Worship*[41] by Buddy Reeve, is a valuable and imaginative resource for use in care homes.
- *Worshiping with Dementia*[42] is a book of meditations, scriptures and prayers edited by Louise Morse.
- *The Gift of Years. Bible reflections for older people.*[43]

When praying with those with dementia, use familiar words that will echo:

> *Our Father which art in heaven, hallowed be thy name.*
>
> *Matthew 6:9 (KJV)*

See the simple prayer overleaf to read, pray and share.

Often, close prayer with a blessing and invite all to join in:

> *The grace of the Lord Jesus Christ, the love of God, and the fellowship of the Holy Spirit be with us all.*
>
> *2 Corinthians 13:13 (GNT)*

If you cannot think of the right words, do not worry because we are told that God's Spirit can help us if we get stuck for words!

> *In certain ways we are weak, but the Spirit is here to help us. For example, when we don't know what to pray for, the Spirit prays for us in ways that cannot be put into words.*
>
> *Romans 8:26 (CEV)*

---

41 B. Reeve; *50 Services of Christian Worship*, PARCHE (Eastbourne).

42 L. Morse (Editor); *Worshiping with Dementia;* Monarch (2010).

43 Jennifer Bute; *The Gift of Years. Bible reflections for older people. January-April 2017;* Bible Reading Fellowship (Abingdon).

A PRAYER FOR THOSE LIVING WITH DEMENTIA, AND FOR ALL OF US

Lord God, I am afraid,
  I cannot understand what is happening
  and what people say.
Lord, I feel lost,
  even after years of living here,
  the place seems strange and frightening.
Lord, I feel isolated and alone,
  even my loved ones sometimes appear to be strangers.
Lord, I feel hopeless and helpless,
  after a lifetime of being able to help others.
Lord, I feel stupid,
  I cannot answer questions
  or even think of how to ask for help.
Lord, I feel humiliated,
  I was so capable,
  but now I cannot even look after myself.
Lord, I feel so dependent,
  even for little things,
  and I was so proud of my independence.

Lord, will I lose you too?
  I forget how to pray,
  but I know I still love you and need you.
Lord, in my fear, my lostness, isolation,
  helplessness, stupidity, humiliation and dependence,
  I cast myself on you.
Holy Spirit, draw near,
  befriend, cover and embrace my soul,
  for I am your child now and for ever.
Jesus said, "Let the children come,"
  so, Lord, let me be with you now and always.

Amen.

PRAYER FOR CARERS AND THE CARED FOR

Lord, in weakness or in strength we bear your image.
We pray for those we love who now live
in a land of shadows
Where the light of memory is dimmed,
Where the familiar lies unknown,
Where the beloved become as strangers;
Hold them in your everlasting arms.

And grant to those who care
A strength to serve,
A patience to persevere,
A love to last and
A peace that passes human understanding.
Hold us in your everlasting arms
Today and for all eternity
Through Jesus Christ our Lord. Amen.

Rt. Rev. James Jones of Liverpool

MEDITATION AND MINDFULNESS

Meditation is not clearing or emptying the mind while sitting cross legged and murmuring "Ommmmmm…" The meditation we need is that of focusing the mind on God and his word: the written word and the living word. This meditation and mindfulness come from the Judeo-Christian tradition but there is no need to be a priest, a rabbi, a monk, a nun or a saint.

Take a portion of scripture and turn it over and over in your mind. Repeat it; think of its meaning and its message for you. Take it into your heart. Remember what God has done for you. Be thankful for the life he has given you and be thankful for this present moment in time. Thank God for your life here and now; this banishes regrets for the past and fears for the future.

David's psalms and the words of Jesus give many verses to focus on. Find a few, memorise, use and make them your own!

The Lord is my light and my salvation; whom shall I fear? The Lord is.the strength of my life; of whom shall I be afraid?

Psalm 27:1 (NIV)

Praise the Lord, O my soul; all my inmost being, praise his holy name. Praise the Lord, O my soul, and forget not all his benefits...

Psalm 103:1-2 (NIV)

Jesus said, "I give you peace, the kind of peace that only I can give. It isn't like the peace that this world can give. So don't be worried or afraid."

John 12:27 (CEV)

Here is an ancient and simple prayer that has been used for centuries for meditation. Repeat it slowly as you breathe in and then out:

"Lord Jesus Christ, Son of God, have mercy on me (a sinner)."[44]

This acknowledges the supremacy and lordship of Jesus Christ. It declares that I am in need of redemption and this is found in Christ alone.

RITUALS AND REMINDERS

Simple actions and objects can sometimes carry and sustain deep messages: of hope, or light, or love, or commitment, or reassurance. These can be valuable in strengthening the faith when memory is failing.

Before his death and resurrection, Jesus had a special meal with his disciples and friends. This action, especially the sharing in bread and wine, was symbolic of his love and sacrifice. Its deep significance to all who follow him is re-enacted as a reminder of

---

[44] *The Way of a Pilgrim;* translated from the Russian by R.M. French; Bantam Doubleday Dell Publishers (1999). The words of the prayer are based on Luke 18:13.

the way of redemption. He asked us to do this to remember him. It is a powerful reminder and blessing.

- Seek and take opportunities to share in Communion, the Lord's Supper.
- Talk of Jesus as the light of the world and a light in times of darkness. Light a candle (or a small night light) and leave it, safely, with your friend.
- Speak and share the words, "Walk in the light,"[45] spoken by Jesus.
- Talk of Mary anointing Jesus' feet with perfume as a symbol of deep devotion, and light or dip an incense stick and leave it so the fragrance lingers. Where it is appropriate, touch the forehead of a special friend with a spot of cologne or perfume.
  May the fragrance of Jesus fill your life.
- Give small piece of a fleece to be held and stroked while talking of the Good Shepherd caring for his sheep in dangerous places.
  May the Good Shepherd find you, hold you, and carry you safely.
- Give a small wooden cross or embroidered cross to hold in the hand and keep when you talk of some aspect of the Passion and the Easter story.
  May the redeeming love of Jesus cleanse and refresh you today.

With any of these messages, recite or sing familiar hymns and songs that carry the same messages and will echo in the mind and memory:

- *Jesus bids us shine* or *Shine, Jesus, shine.*
- *May the fragrance of Jesus fill this place.*
- *The Lord's my Shepherd, I'll not want.*
- *Jesus Christ is risen today, Alleluia!*

[45] See John 8:12; 11:9.

The Cross in My Hand

I hold this small cross in my hand
A simple reminder to me
Of the fact that I am a Christian
No matter where I may be.

It reminds me too, to be thankful
For my blessings day by day
And to live my thanks quite clearly
In all that I do and say.

It's also a daily reminder
Of the peace and comfort I share
With all who know my Lord Jesus
And give themselves to his care.

Anon.

"FEAR NOT" – JESUS' FAVOURITE WORD OF ENCOURAGEMENT

It is translated differently in different places. Here is a powerful passage:

Jesus said to his disciples, "Don't be worried!
Have faith in God and have faith in me.
There are many rooms in my Father's house. I wouldn't tell you this, unless it was true. I am going there to prepare a place for each of you."

John 14:1-2 (CEV)

He goes on in the same speech to say:

"I give you peace, the kind of peace that only I can give. It isn't like the peace that this world can give. So don't be worried or afraid."

John 14:27 (CEV)

Jesus gives powerful promises, but they are especially relevant to those who suffer from dementia. Take a firm hold on this assurance, endorse it for yourself, your loved ones and those you care for.

Then feel his promised peace.

In Lighter Mode: God's Word, Good Therapy

Blessed is the one who does not walk in step with the wicked or stand in the way that sinners take or sit in the company of mockers, but whose delight is in the law of the LORD, and who meditates on his law day and night. That person is like a tree planted by streams of water, which yields its fruit in season and whose leaf does not wither – whatever they do prospers.

Psalm 1 (NIV)

At the worship service in the Home for Seniors, one of the residents was asked to read Psalm 1. She stumbled on one word and read, "...who medicates on his law day and night."
The whole group roared with laughter. Laughter was truly their medication that day!

Laughter is the medication that we all need.

A cheerful heart is good medicine, but a crushed spirit dries up the bones.

Proverbs 17:22 (NIV)

In Lighter Mode: Learn a New Language

Learning a new language is said to be good exercise for the brain, but in fact most Seniors have learnt a new language in recent years! There are a host of new words, but here are new meanings to old words and phrases:

'Fast food' was what you ate in Lent, a 'Big Mac' was an oversized raincoat and 'crumpet' we had toasted for tea. The 'pill' was a simple medicinal tablet, not a liberating, demographic-changing contraceptive. A 'chip' was a piece of wood or fried potato, 'hardware' meant nuts and bolts and 'software' wasn't a word. 'Digital' was to do with fingers and toes, not with numbers, music or images! 'Sheltered accommodation' was where you waited for a bus.

'Partners' was a business term. We 'courted' before computer dating, got married first and then lived together (sounds quaint but usually worked). 'Making out' referred to how you did in your exams. 'Stud' was something that fastened a collar to a shirt. 'Going all the way' meant staying on the bus to the terminus. For us, 'time sharing' meant togetherness.

Before 1940, 'Rock Music' was a mother's lullaby, 'Eldorado' was an ice-cream, a 'gay person' was the life and soul of the party. 'AIDS' just meant beauty treatment or help for someone in trouble. In our day, 'grass' was mown, 'coke' was kept in the coalhouse, a 'joint' was a piece of meat you ate on Sundays and 'pot' was something you cooked in. Lies were lies, not 'post truth'!

CHAPTER FIVE

Preparing to Manage Dementia

The following sections are mainly directed to the family and the personal carers for someone with dementia. Others are directly for the person with dementia. If the language appears ambiguous, change the sense to your own situation. It is intended to be positive and helpful!

The limitations and the possibilities for management

There is currently no drug that can cure the condition.[46] A few medicines may slow the progress of the disease, but these may also produce undesirable side effects.[47]

Despite this – and this is important – there are many things that *can* be done to live well with the condition. These include physical exercise, cognitive behavioral treatment, social contacts, music, brain exercises, spiritual support and an appropriate diet. There is now good evidence that regular, vigorous physical exercise can not only slow dementia, but can actually bring some improvement.[48]

Although memory and understanding fail, feelings remain and may be intensified, especially anxiety and fear. These feelings can

[46] Rev. Dr. Joanna Collicutt; *Thinking of you;* Bible Reading Fellowship (Abingdon, 2017).

[47] See the section entitled 'The role of medicines' on page 122.

[48] See page 111 and 184.

be helped with an appropriate action and words; for example, they respond to reassurance, comfort and love. You might feel that because your friend no longer remembers your name or the experiences you shared, it is not worth talking, but there is evidence that sharing music or pictures that are important to you both can calm fears. A warm hug, a gentle, appropriate touch and a few words that show affection can reduce anxiety and give comfort.

This is such an important matter and an opportunity for positive action.[49]

A patient-centred care for all those with dementia

A core recommendation for management is the concept of Patient Centred Care (PCC) for all those with dementia.

This approach was developed by Professor Tom Kitwood. It is based on "the ethic that all human beings are of absolute value and are worthy of respect, no matter their disability" and "the conviction that people with dementia can live fulfilling lives".[50]

In practice this depends on the simple Bible-based principle summarised by Jesus:

> *Do to others whatever you would like them to do to you. This is the essence of all that is taught in the law and the prophets.*
>
> *Matthew 7:12 (NLT)*

> *Treat someone with dementia in the way that you would like to be treated if you had dementia.*

---

[49] See page 116.

[50] Kitwood T.; *Building up the mosaic of good practice;* J. Dementia Care (1996):3:12-13.

This means we should:

- Care for the whole person, not concentrate on the diseased brain.
- Use and enhance the abilities and emotions that the person still has, and not concentrate on what has been lost and is not functioning.
- Manage the person, so far as is possible, in their natural context: their family, marriage, cultural setting etc.

Care-giving in dementia attempts to hold the person together. It involves compassion, comfort, inclusion, attachment, occupation, a sense of identity and, for Christians, love in the spirit of Christ. Tom Kitwood declared, "It might be said that there is only one all-encompassing need – the need for love."

A special and practical application of PCC is 'Comfortable Dementia' or the SPECAL method.[51] It starts with learning from the patient what is or has been most important in his or her life. This is their 'Primary Theme' which will be their most enduring memories and the most important focus for them as a person, their identity.[52]

Build circles of support and join helpful networks

Dementia not only damages the neurones, the nerve cells of the brain, but ultimately destroys all the relationships of the individual. Slowly and progressively, as social skills and memory decline, the circles of contact will gradually fall away. Social isolation and loneliness are real. Eventually the close family and designated carers will be the only ones left, and they too are in danger of being isolated from the community.

| *Strengthen the links. Build the support.* |

---

[51] Oliver James; *Contented Dementia;* Vermilion, Ebony Publishing (2008).
[52] The SPECAL method is described more fully on page 153.

The family, friends and close carers of someone with dementia must deliberately reach out and build links to other groups and build circles of support around the person with dementia. Unfortunately fear of the condition and feelings of shame may make people withdraw. It is a shock when even the near and dear are not recognised.

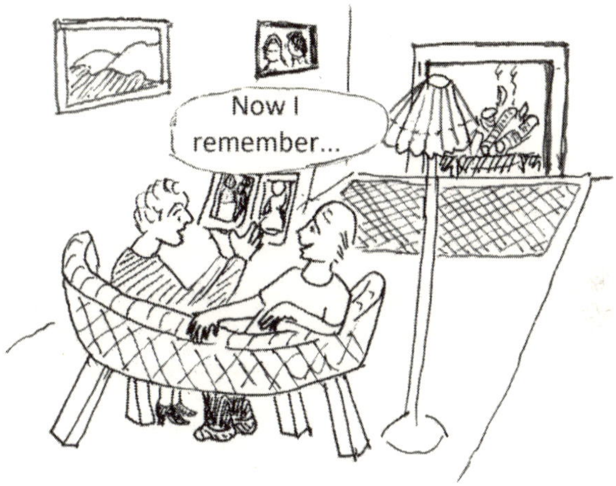

*"Ah, our wedding pictures.
Now I remember who we are!"*

Much help will be needed during the dementia journey. Start to strengthen ties to all 'loved ones', the family and friends. In addition to the statutory medical and social services, contact the Alzheimer's Society, ageUK, any church with a dementia-friendly team, brain-boosting clubs, chair-based exercise groups and others who may be helpful. Even in early stages of dementia, reach out for help and strengthen links.

When dementia comes into a home, work hard to counter the tendency for shy reticence. Encourage boldness to speak out about real needs and ask for help. Encourage the individual and the family to chat and be friendly, even when they are nervous and fearful. It can be hard, but many others have been down this road and have discovered organisations and people who can help them.

The first circle of support is often the family. They will be sad and nervous, not knowing what to expect. But encourage regular phoning, visiting and, if possible, do things together: shopping, going to church, walking, attending family events and visiting others. Family will also be important to help with planning for the future, filling in forms and giving essential emotional support. Making proper legal arrangements for decisions and finances should be considered earlier rather than later.

Support from individual friends or from a group can sometimes be as important as family. Visits, outings, practical help and emotional support are all vital.[53]

If the person with dementia is a member of the church, this fellowship can be very important: accompanying them to church, sitting with them and praying with them when appropriate. Reassure them that though they may forget things and people, God will never forget them. Some churches have a team whose purpose is to make the place feel dementia-friendly.[54]

Support from the Health Team is essential. A sympathetic GP who listens carefully and keeps you as healthy as possible is a good start. However, he or she should be able to point you to health, social and voluntary services that will be a great asset. Nurses from the Memory clinics, the Alzheimer's Society and other organisations are wonderful.[55]

The Social Services in UK give both statutory and practical help for those with dementia, so it is necessary to learn what they can provide. This will be different in different geographic areas. Sometimes there is a contact person, or this person may be from the Alzheimer's Society or another independent charity, who will tell you what help is available and give telephone contact numbers. They will draw up a care plan according to individual needs and, depending on the circumstances, may help provide it.

---

[53] See section entitled 'Visiting someone with dementia' on page 102.

[54] See the section entitled 'A dementia-friendly church and community' on page 68.

[55] See the list of useful resources on page 96.

They can also inform about what is available from the independent charitable side. This includes not only activities related directly to dementia, assessment of a person with dementia, their condition, assessment for Attendance Allowance and services like memory clubs and 'Singing for the Brain', but also things related to general health and wellbeing.

KATE'S STORY

Janet had moderate Alzheimer's disease. Her daughter Kate was her main carer and worked hard to get all the services coordinated.

> *It is amazing all that is available to help me care for my mum. I used to be PA for an important CEO of a busy company. I need all my skills to organise things for Mum!*

Safeguarding and planning ahead

Melissa's story below contains two strands of planning ahead and protection. One regards financial protection when a person loses mental capacity, as with dementia, and the other is protection from unwanted medical interventions at the end of life. These matters concern not only the individual, but also the family and close friends. They should be thought about and openly discussed long before action is needed in a medical emergency or at the end of life. This section is helpful both for those living with dementia and also those who are concerned about planning for 'a good death'. That is something we would all like, so it is a plea that we do not postpone thinking, talking and planning for it!

MELISSA'S STORY

Melissa was the only child of an elderly couple, Robert and Agnes. They both died as octogenarians in a single sad year. Robert had a bad heart with angina, pain in the chest when he walked uphill.

One night he had the pain even in bed. Early next morning, Agnes heard him call out and then found him blue and unresponsive. She panicked and called Melissa who lived two hours away.

Melissa said, "Quick, dial 999 and tell them he has chest pain."

The man in the ambulance call centre was helpful but directive. "If you cannot feel a pulse, pull him out of bed onto the floor on his back and I will tell you what to do. Is he breathing? No? Still no pulse? Press hard on his chest forty times a minute. Right; press, release, press, release. Keep going."

The paramedics were fast, but still it was the longest ten minutes of Agnes' life. They took over resuscitation but much more vigorously. There was a nasty crack noise from Robert's chest. With the defibrillator shock they got his heart started and then it was a blue-light chase to A&E.

Sadly, Robert never recovered consciousness. Because his heart had been stopped for some time, he later had a stroke from which he died five days later. Robert was not the only one who died from the traumatic treatment. Agnes never recovered, and within a couple of months died of progressive frailty. Another consequence was that Melissa vowed that she would never permit any resuscitation on herself! She checked the legislation and wrote for herself an Advance Decision or 'Living Will' that clearly instructed "no resuscitation" if she had a heart attack.

After the traumatic year of her parent's death, Melissa's life took off. She had been the competent PA to the manager of a successful stationery business for nearly twenty years. She was an amateur artist, and left the company to run her own business of making and selling an attractive brand of birthday and other cards. Business was blooming and her eye-catching cards were popular, even used by celebrities.

She had just turned sixty when she had a fall and broke her leg badly and the medical report stated she had progressive osteoporosis, weak and fragile bones. Within a couple of years she was almost immobilised and imprisoned in her bungalow with severe pain. She had no relatives except a cousin, Bronwyn, in rural Wales. Fortunately, her friendly neighbour Izzi took her bank card and helped her with supermarket shopping each week.

Over a couple of years, in addition to her immobility, Melissa developed significant and progressive dementia. She could not cope with her birthday card business and finances. She was constantly losing things. If it had not been for her friend Izzi's stepson Derek, who came to her rescue, her affairs would have been impossible. Then the payment for her utility bills started to bounce and her bank card ceased to work. Bronwyn and her husband arrived from Wales to help her find a care home. They discovered that her savings accounts had been completely emptied and Derek had left home. His stepmother Izzi had no idea where he was. Sadly, it was a classic case of dementia defrauded.

DON'T BE PANICKED!

Most people, when they hear the words, "I am sorry to tell you that you have early dementia," feel a flood of fear flow into their minds. Among the serious thoughts are these:

- "When my brain gets worse, who will look after me when I cannot look after myself?"
- "Who will decide things for me when I can no longer decide for myself or cannot communicate what I want?"
- "Who will look after my money matters?"
- "Who will help me decide about medical conditions and treatments?"
- "Who will protect me from physical abuse and financial fraudsters?"

Try to stay calm. You are not alone. Others have walked this path and there are signposts, legislation, organisations and, most important, friends to help you on the journey.

First, remember to take courage and travel with hope. Often dementia may move very slowly and there can be years of good and happy living after the diagnosis.

Second, be assured that there are many things that can be done and many organisations to help you deal with your situation.

Third, there are practical and legal provisions to protect you from harm or from being given treatments you do not want. There are statutory mechanisms you can set up to protect yourself from harm or exploitation.

In Melissa's situation she should have appointed Bronwyn as attorney for both finances and for health and welfare. Now look at the issues.

PLAN AHEAD – BUT START NOW

While you are still able to think about your future, talk to others, especially trusted friends and close members of your family, and plan ahead. Do this as soon as you can and make decisions and plans about your future care and finances, or those of a loved one.

These discussions and choices are important. Do not delay by denying that there is anything wrong or by thinking, "I'm alright now; I can do these things later." The best time to act is now, while your thinking is still good.

PROTECTION AND CARE FOR THOSE WITH DEMENTIA

People with dementia often become unable to make decisions for themselves as their condition progresses. When this happens, the person is said to 'lack capacity'. Dementia is one of several possible reasons for a lack of capacity. That is a legal term, but remember that the person is still a loved and valued human being!

In UK there are laws that protect such people, for example, The Mental Capacity Act in England and Wales. (There are similar laws for Scotland and Northern Ireland.) This law protects your right to make your own decisions and be involved in, and get support for, any decisions that affect you. If a person lacks capacity, any decisions taken on their behalf must be in their best interests. It must always be assumed that everyone is able to make a decision for themselves, until it is proven that they cannot.

Mental capacity is the ability to make decisions for yourself. Assessing capacity uses information from the individual, the family, carers and professionals. It can be quite a complicated legal business, so it is good to start early on, especially if you do not have a close relative who can help with this.

This book is not the right place to explain all of this process, but this chapter will explain some of the words used in relation to protection and tell you and your carers where to find the information you will need to set up good protection for yourself, your health, wellbeing and finances.

DECISION-MAKING AND MENTAL CAPACITY

A person who has capacity should be able to understand relevant information and retain it long enough to make decisions. They should be able to weigh up the information, make a decision and communicate it to others by one means or another.

Capacity may change over time, coming and going. We all know we can think better when we are fresh and fit, compared with when we are tired and ill. A person may have capacity for some sorts of decisions, what to eat and wear, but not more complicated things like financial or medical decisions.

As capacity declines, personal carers will be able to help with simple day by day decisions. For more complicated decisions, people with family or appropriate links and specialist knowledge may be appointed through a legal process. They are called attorneys and cover two separate areas: either finances or health and welfare issues.

APPOINTMENT OF SPECIAL DECISION MAKERS – ATTORNEYS

The Mental Capacity Act enables a person to choose and appoint an individual or several people to take decisions for them if in the future they cannot make decisions for themselves. The intention is that these attorneys will make decisions in line with what the client would like and what is in their best interest, even when they cannot decide or communicate these views. Someone with early dementia does not have to appoint someone if they do not want to.

Choosing attorneys is a vital decision. An attorney should be over 18 and not a paid care worker. They must always act in your best interests. The attorney should be an appropriate person for the type of decision or action. For important medical treatment decisions, a medical or paramedical professional would be more appropriate, or an attorney could take appropriate advice from such professionals. For financial and property issues, someone with understanding of finances, property commerce and legal procedures may be a good attorney.

Think carefully about whom to give the power to.

Consider these questions about possible attorneys:

- Are the people you wish to appoint willing to be appointed?
- Can you trust them to act in your best interests?
  Talk to family and close friends; tell them what you plan and why.
- Do you want to consider more than one attorney?
- Are there likely to be any disagreements or problems between them?
- Do you want different attorneys to be appointed for different things?
  This can be specified in the agreement.
- Do you wish to limit the attorney's authority (for example, financial accountability)?
- Do they handle their own money well?

- Do you think they understand your wishes and feelings about your money and your health, treatments and beliefs?
- If you have strong views on a particular type of treatment, are they aware of this?
- Do they know you well enough to take your views into account when deciding what is in your best interests?
- Do they understand your beliefs, views or feelings; and would you trust them to take these into account when making decisions?

Setting up a Lasting Power of Attorney (LPA) is the legal method that enables someone to choose whom they would wish to make decisions for them in future if they become unable to make decisions themselves. The person or persons they appoint will then become their attorney.

To make a LPA an application form must be completed, then correctly signed, witnessed and dated. Finally, it must be registered with the Office of the Public Guardian before it can be used.

There are two different types of LPA, each relating to different decisions. Someone can have both types, but will needs two sets of forms.

- *LPA for property and financial affairs* – this gives the attorney (or attorneys) the power to make decisions about the person's financial and property matters, such as selling a house or managing a bank account.
- *LPA for health and welfare* – this gives the attorney (or attorneys) the power to make decisions about the person's health and personal welfare, such as day-to-day care, medical treatment or where they should live.

Most important decisions are around the need to increase help in the home or move the person to a care home.

WHO MAKES DECISIONS FOR SOMEONE WHO LACKS MENTAL CAPACITY?

If someone with dementia can still make simple decisions, their opinion and wishes must be accepted so long as these are safe for the individual.

After capacity is lost:

- *Everyday decisions about washing, dressing, eating or activities:* whoever is with the person at the time can make these decisions, for example, the carer, family or care worker.
- *Decisions about the person's finances or property:* their attorney or deputy for property and financial affairs will make these decisions.
- *Decisions about where the person will live and receive care:* if they have an attorney or deputy for health and welfare, they can make the decision; if not, a professional such as a social worker or doctor will make the decision.
- *Decisions relating to life-sustaining treatment:* if the person appointed an attorney for health and welfare, then they may be able to make the decision; if not, then it will be an appropriate doctor or consultant.

WILLS

Everyone should make a will. It allows you to choose who will inherit your money and your possessions. It is simpler to set up than a LPA. Indeed, you can write a few sentences about whom you want to receive what when you die and get two responsible adults to witness your signature and add their addresses and date. If your affairs are more complicated, you should consult a solicitor or ask someone to help you download a simple will from the internet.

ADVANCE DECISION AND ADVANCE VALUES STATEMENT

Regarding what is important to you, you may think that your own family know how you would like to be treated and what are the things that you value most in life. However, it is a good to think about these things and to write them down. You may simply write down your priorities and preferences, your likes and dislikes; dietary and clothing preferences, music desires, religious and other beliefs and how you would like to be cared for in a terminal illness or even after death. This can be used if in the future you are not in a position to state your wishes.

It is a good idea to give this to family, close friends and also those involved in caring for you. If you have no family, or even close friends, you may give it to your family doctor who should act responsibly in carrying out your hopes.

This simple document should be considered by those looking after you and determining what is in your best interest, even though it is not legally binding.

ADVANCE DECISION ABOUT MEDICAL TREATMENT – A LIVING WILL

If you feel strongly that there are some medical treatments you would not want to receive in certain circumstances, you should write this down.

This will only be used if you lose your capacity to make or communicate decisions, for example, if you are unconscious or have severe dementia. It is not used to deny basic care like giving pain relief, water or food.

It is sensible to discuss such a decision with your family doctor and members of your family.

A written Advance Decision is legally binding and must be followed. One specific decision is a “Do Not Resuscitate” order, a specific request not to have your heart or breathing restarted if they stop. An example of such a form is shown overleaf. This is the form that Melissa wrote for herself after the traumatic death of her father. (This version is most suitable for someone with a recent diagnosis of dementia, or worried about dementia, and with other health problems. If the wording is not quite right for you, you can add or delete information. Look at the other versions on the ADA website: *www.ADassistance.org.uk.* If you have any questions, phone 01757 289453 in UK.)

A Living Will is a written advance decision to refuse treatment and be treated in a specific way in certain circumstances. It will only be used in situations if there comes a time when you lack capacity to make or communicate your decisions.

Useful resources

www.gov.uk/government/uploads/system/uploads/attachment_data/file/497253/Mental-capacity-act-code-of-practice.pdf

The dementia guide
Alzheimer's Society (2016)
www.alzheimers.org.uk

Powers of attorney
ageUK (2016)
www.ageuk.org.uk/moneymatters

Advance Decisions Assistance (ADA)
www.adassistance.org.uk/contact-us
(01757) 289453
ADA c/o Professor Celia Kitzinger, Department of Sociology,
University of York, York, YO10 5DD
info@ADassistance.org.uk

ADVANCE DECISION FORM

(Based on Version D from ADA)

This Advance Decision is intended to apply indefinitely unless I specifically revoke it.
I give permission for anyone legitimately involved in my care to read it.

Your name (block capitals):

____

Your address:

____

____

____

Your date of birth: __________________________

Your NHS no. (if known): _______________________

GP's name & address:

____

____

____

<u>Statement for you to sign:</u>

When I am unable to make or communicate decisions about my medical treatment, I wish to REFUSE all treatments or interventions which may prolong my life.

This refusal includes (but is not limited to):

- Cardio-pulmonary resuscitation (CPR)
- Ventilation
- Treatments designed to replace a vital bodily function (e.g. heart pacemaker)
- A feeding tube

- Antibiotics given for a potentially life-threatening infection
- Specialised treatments for particular conditions (such as chemotherapy, dialysis)
- Other current treatments/medications (if relevant) - say what these are:

____

____

I maintain this refusal even if it shortens my life.
If I refuse food and/or drink by mouth, I refuse repeated attempts to feed/hydrate me; or being persuaded or cajoled to eat or drink - even if this refusal shortens my life.

I do consent to treatment to alleviate pain or distress, even if it shortens my life.

Your signature: ____________________ Date: __________

Witness' signature: _________________ Date: __________

Witness' name & address:

____

(Delete note below if you have NOT been diagnosed with dementia.)

<u>Important note:</u> Because I have recently been diagnosed with dementia, I have attached a statement from a health practitioner confirming that at the time of completing this Advance Decision, I have the mental capacity to make the decisions contained in it.

<u>Advance Values Statement:</u>
You may choose to include a further short statement here to explain the decisions you have made and what is important to you. This may be helpful to those looking after you.

MELISSA'S ADVANCE VALUES STATEMENT

Below is an example, based on Melissa's story from page 87.

I am writing this Advance Decision in order to plan for the future, as best I can. I have recently been diagnosed with dementia (Alzheimer's disease), and know that this will get worse. For as long as possible, I hope to lead a full life and I should like to die at home, in my own bed, if possible. I do not want to be rushed into hospital in my final hours.

The things that are important to me are my independence, my social life, my church, and family life, especially with my niece Bronwyn and her children. When I am no longer able to look after myself, I do not want to move to Wales to live with Bronwyn and her children. (When my Aunt Alice got Alzheimer's disease and stayed with her daughter, it was so hard that it nearly split the family.)

I am filled with horror at the prospect of moving into a care home with all the restrictions, but if I am helpless I accept that there may be no other way.

However, I have a number of other health problems - high blood pressure, angina, and heart arrhythmia - so I am at high risk of having a stroke or heart attack. I have written my Advance Decision to refuse all treatments for these conditions, including resuscitation. My hope is that I may die sooner of a heart attack or stroke than slowly from dementia. In case I do not die of a heart attack or stroke, I have also refused the treatments and interventions that are common in late-stage dementia: antibiotics and a feeding tube.

I know what I want to happen and I am settled in these wishes.

<u>Important note:</u> Because I have recently been diagnosed with dementia (Alzheimer's Disease), I have attached a statement from my GP confirming that at the time of completing this Advance Decision, I have the mental capacity to make the decisions contained in it.

Melissa's signature & date

____

Witness' signature & date

____

In Lighter Mode: Name Dropping

Forgetting the names of people you know quite well is common when you get older. It leads to funny situations. Never be afraid to say to someone, "Please remind me of your name. I know you so well, but your name has just slipped me." Everyone will understand your predicament.

Her Majesty Queen Elizabeth's picture is on every postage stamp, coin and paper money note in UK.
She told of her visit to a retirement home. She is really good at chatting with all sorts of people, but she was finding conversation with one old resident rather difficult. So she asked the elderly lady, "Do you know who I am?"
The old resident replied, "Don't worry about it, my dear. Just ask the nurse when she comes around, and she will tell you who you are!"

In Lighter Mode: Personal Memory Aid

"Hey, John, how was the memory clinic that you have been attending?"

"It was great, Mike, and made a big difference. They use handy psychological techniques, visualisation, association and so on. Really helps me to remember things."

"That's good. I may need to use the place. What is the name of the clinic?"

"Oh, just let me use one top technique I learnt there. What is the name of that lovely flower with the perfume and the sharp thorns?"

"Would it be 'rose'?"

"Yes, that's it... Rose, what is the name of the memory clinic?"

Note: The most effective memory aid is a live spouse.

CHAPTER SIX

Practical Steps to Cope with Dementia

Visiting someone with dementia

This can be more valuable than you think. Often visitors, both family and friends, feel awkward because they do not understand the condition and cannot communicate normally. Genuine friendly concern and warmth is what matters; it is not about any special technique. There is evidence that visits have meaning, even to those who do not show any obvious response.

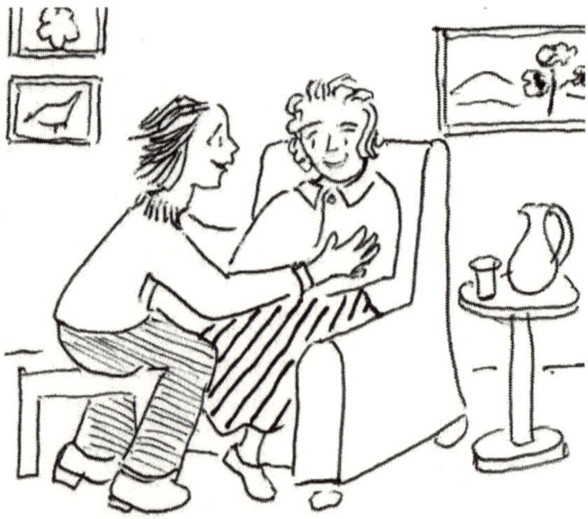

Empathy and physical contact are most valued and remembered!

If you do not know the person, find out as much about them as possible before you visit. If possible, ask their family and carers about their childhood and what was important to the person, not just the recent medical history. Did they have special hobbies, interests or experiences that they may remember and could start a conversation in which they would be happy to engage?

Those who have dementia may have trouble recognizing people, but they can have feelings of anxiety, fear, depression and loneliness. These feelings often remain even though their memories are failing. They may also retain spiritual awareness. Visits can stimulate warm feelings, bring comfort and reaffirm spiritual truths.

Communicating effectively

Dr Jennifer Bute gives the following recommendations:

> *I have had the privilege of looking after others with dementia, so after I had been diagnosed with Alzheimer's Dementia ... I was able to anticipate the problems ... the person with dementia is still there, trapped inside the disease ...*
>
> *I passionately believe that care can be more proactive than is usually the case ... when the front door (to my brain) is shut and the key is lost there is usually a back door or a ladder with which to climb in the window. Those who care about the trapped person might like a few tools to help make 'escape routes'!*
>
> *Advice to those with dementia: be bold, and tell people you meet –*
>
> - *If I don't recognise you, please remind me who you are and in what context I know you and, if necessary, give me additional clues.*

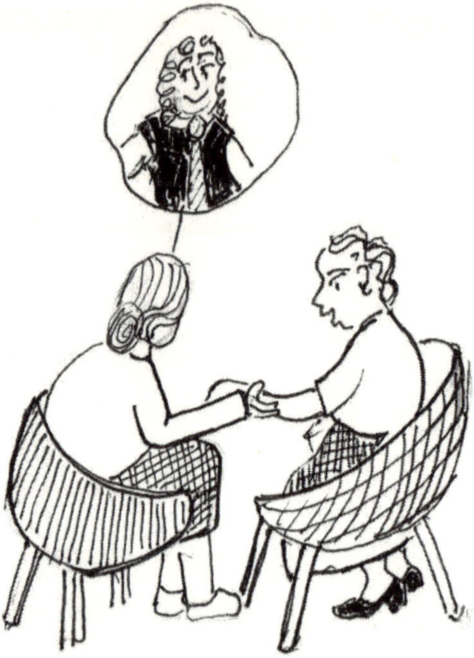

"Ah, now I remember – you are my little sister. But you used to have a gym tunic and pigtails."

- *If you tell me about something important, or remind me of anything, please also email me. I can then review the information, with help if necessary, to make sense of it. (Many people with dementia will not be able to use email so perhaps simply write things down.)*
- *If I look lost or bewildered, I probably am. Please help me if possible or direct me to a safe place or contact my husband (or carer).*
- *Some days I can communicate more easily and can talk quite coherently. I tend to be at my best in the mornings.*

Additional tips when visiting and helping those with dementia –

- *Wear something bright or colourful; it's more memorable and cheerful.*
- *Approach from the front; don't tap on the back or shoulder.*
- *Always introduce yourself with your name and a simple explanation. Possibly say where we met before and what is our connection.*
- *Smile and make eye contact.*
- *Sit at the same level.*
- *Perhaps touch their hand if appropriate.*
- *Avoid choices, preferably offer one item! A cup of tea? Not, "Tea, coffee or chocolate?" but, "Let us get tea and your favourite biscuits?"*
- *Simplify and calm the environment.*
- *Remove or reduce stress triggers; noise, bright lights, too many people.*
- *Involve them in activities where possible. Don't stop them doing something because they aren't doing it 'properly'.*
- *Don't exclude them from conversations; they often understand more than you realise. Response may be slow.*
- *If the person seems stressed or unresponsive, change to a familiar activity, make a cup of tea together, go for a walk or a car ride.*
- *Music can calm and reassure.*

- *When words fail, an appropriate touch or hug can reassure. Fear is less frightening when you hold hands.*
- *Talk about hobbies, passions, things that meant a lot when they were younger.*
- *Look at pictures, videos, DVDs of events, outings or holidays.*
- *With any activity, ask, "Is this a problem for them or for me, and who can adapt more easily?"*
- *Controlling is not the same as caring.*

Jennifer Bute also says:

Remember that for me, Jesus has always been my centre.

CONVERSATION IS GOOD

- Speak simply, clearly, one comment at a time. Many older people are hard of hearing. Help them with their hearing aids and batteries if necessary.
- Be positive and reassuring.
- Avoid questions if possible.
- Listen and give time for answers or comments.
- Listen for the meaning behind the words people use or stories they tell:
    - "Are you cold?" – Is she actually saying, "I am not really enjoying this."?
    - "What is the time?" – Perhaps, "I have no idea what I'm meant to be doing…"
    - "Is it getting dark yet?" – Perhaps, "How long does it take to get back home?"
    - "I must go home now," might mean, "I am feeling lost or uncomfortable."

- Stories – The stories people tell may have a deeper meaning. There was a woman at a day centre who repeatedly told of her first day at school when she wet herself and felt humiliated by the teacher and everyone laughed. She may have been indicating that this is how she felt now.
- Acknowledge the emotions behind the words that are spoken.
- Accept incorrect statements as they may be caused by memory loss or faulty logic. Don't make corrections or denials.
- Repetition, repetition, repetition -- This may be an attempt to talk or get your attention. Learn to love not hate questions. Give reassuring answers and don't be embarrassed about repeating the same answer.
- Be patient. If there is no response, sometimes holding hands or an appropriate touch will be the most meaningful communication.

BE READY FOR QUESTIONS ABOUT ABSENT PEOPLE.

Jennifer Bute says:

If a person asks where is someone who has died, you can say – "He is not here at the moment, so let's have a cup of tea."

You may give an understandable reason of why they are not here now. For example, if Stanley (my late husband) is absent, you could remind me that he often used to be away working in Africa. If you say, "You know he is dead!" it causes a sudden panic and grief! Divert, there is no need to tell lies.

She also observes:

> *When my mind is 'adrift' and 'I'm living in a different time' I may think that some people are not yet born or married, or are someone else.*

AFFIRMING MOMENTS

Take every opportunity to give encouragement:

- "You always were good at jigsaws..." (even if the present one has a limited number of pieces).
- "You were always good with pencils and colours..." (even if the only books you now use are children's colouring in books).

Smile, and share a simple joke. Laugh whenever possible. It's a tonic!

Here are some suggestions of things to take or do:

- Take a picture magazine, postcard or a flower catalogue.
- Play a game – draughts, dominoes, Ludo, Connect Four etc.
- If appropriate, take a soft toy for them to hold or stroke, or a lavender bag.
- Listen to a CD – familiar music, hymns or songs.
- Watch a DVD of flowers, gardens, water views.
- Reminisce about the past, people or places.
- Look at photographs or illustrated books.
- If you are a Christian, ask if they would like you to read a passage from the Bible. It should be in a familiar version for them, possibly the Authorized Version. Read a prayer or creed from the Book of Common Prayer. Say the Lord's prayer.

Departure should not be a 'big deal'. Some care homes recommend, "Parachute in, but evaporate out," a dramatic and announced entry, but a quiet and unobtrusive exit. Simple explanations are accepted: "I'm off to the loo," not, "See you soon!"

You may be distressed by their condition but be encouraged in that you will have lessened their isolation and loneliness by your visit. The visit need not last long; it is the feelings that remain, not the length of time spent. They may well forget that you came, but the warmth and feelings that you care will not be forgotten.

Visiting the vulnerable and incarcerated is a good thing to do. Remember:

> *"Lord, when did we ... see you ill or in prison and go to visit you?" ... The King will reply, "Truly I tell you, whatever you did for one of the least of these brothers and sisters of mine, you did for me."*
>
> *Matthew 25:36,40.*

Involvement in activities brings hope

At present there is no cure for dementia.

The rate at which dementia gets worse is variable, and often quite slow. Therefore there is time for hope, and scope for interventions that really can improve life for those with the condition. Interventions can slow the progression of Alzheimer's disease, and possibly other forms of dementia, and can make life interesting and enjoyable.

Care no longer means simply giving protection. People with dementia must be involved in life as much as possible and be stimulated. Give them the opportunity to work at some tasks and enjoy the aspects of life to which they can respond.

As well as Jennifer Bute, there are other well-known personalities, such as Christine Bryden, who have had dementia for over two decades and are advocates for positive interventions and changing attitudes to the disease.[56]

---

[56] Jennifer Bute; *www.gloriousopportunity.org*
Christine Bryden; *Dancing with Dementia. My story of living positively with dementia;* Jessica Kingsley Publishers (2005).

Also, much can be done to guide and support the carers, those who look after those with dementia over months and years.

Interventions known to help in dementia

These are briefly listed below, but expanded on in the following pages.

- Physical exercise: walking, group exercises to music, swimming etc.
- Mental stimulation: "brain training", especially mental arithmetic, and reading out loud to someone and explaining what you read. Also puzzles, quizzes, card and board games, language learning etc.
- Cognitive behavioural therapy (CBT), which is often combined with other interventions.
- Social interaction: maintain your contacts by visits, memory clubs, a supportive circle of friends of family who keep in touch regularly, dementia-friendly churches etc.
- Historical memory reminders aid recall: photo albums, memory box, autobiography.
- Short-term memory joggers: diary, calendar, journal, big clock, pictures of people, notebook, noticeboard and sticky notes etc.
- Music stimulation: community choir, Playlist for Life, 'desert island' tunes.
- Intergeneration social interaction – and fun!
- Care for pets and plants; interaction and responsibility.
- Spiritual strengthening: church, Bible, prayer and friendship groups.
- Stay involved with your hobbies, handcrafts and gardening.
- Maintain everyday skills; continue simple domestic responsibilities.
- Dietary modifications which might help; a Mediterranean-type diet.

- Medication: general or specific for brain and other systems.
- Combinations of these interventions.

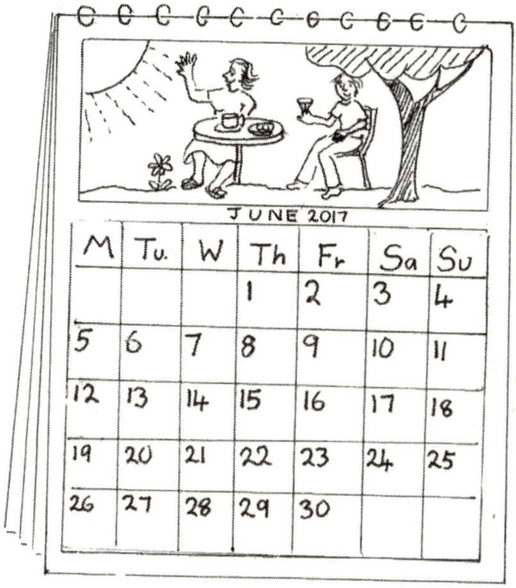

A calendar with space to write in birthdays and appointments. Keep it handy.

PHYSICAL EXERCISE

There is strong evidence that physical exercise benefits those with dementia. It improves cognitive function, practical thinking, and the ability to carry out everyday activities.[57] Regular walking, even short distances, is simple and worthwhile. Exercise carried out regularly in groups, often to the accompaniment of music with social engagement and encouragement, enhances the sense of wellbeing.

---

[57] Northey J.M. et al.; *Exercise interventions for cognitive function in adults older than 50: a systematic review with meta-analysis;* Br J Sports Med (2017); doi:10.1136/bjsports-2016-096587.

Group dancing is valuable for the same reasons and stimulates balance and coordination.

MENTAL STIMULATION, 'BRAIN TRAINING'

As with physical exercise, it is recognised that the "use it or lose it" principle is important for the brain. Unfortunately, those losing their memories may be intimidated by word games, and number games like Sudoku can become boring. Two simple procedures have credible value: reading out loud to someone and explaining what you read, and mental arithmetic.

Crosswords, other puzzles, quizzes, and card and board games which help concentration are useful. Learning a new musical instrument or a new language are good but challenging.

A new generation of simple but engaging electronic games that can catch the interest and be managed by older people is on the horizon. Using electronic tablets and a format that adjusts to the memory level of individuals with cognitive impairment, these new games can hold the attention of Seniors and in a controlled trial have shown "robust improvement in episodic memory".[58] However clever this 'gamification' of brain training, it is an individual method that misses the social component that is discussed on page 116. Playing simple tabletop board games and doing quizzes in groups is stimulating with the additional benefit of a friendly social environment.

COGNITIVE BEHAVIOURAL THERAPY

Cognitive Behavioural Therapy (CBT) is a talking treatment that teaches coping skills to manage your problems. It starts by examining your thoughts, beliefs and attitudes and then changes them to affect the things you do, your attitude and behaviour.

---

[58] Savulich, G. et al.; *Cognitive Training Using a Novel Memory Game on an iPad in Patients with Amnestic Mild Cognitive Impairment (aMCI);* Int J Neuropsychopharmacol (Jul 2017); pyx040. *https://doi.org/10.1093/ijnp/pyx040, July 2017.*

In general terms, CBT is important for those with early dementia because it counters the very negative thinking, the pessimistic media coverage and the fear associated with the diagnosis. The general public, the health professionals and especially those with dementia need to think about this disease in a much more positive way. We know that with encouragement and good support there can be years – possibly *many* years – of good life after diagnosis.

This positive thinking is exactly what Jennifer Bute applied when she was diagnosed with dementia. She said to herself, and to all whom she contacted, "I know a lot about this condition, I helped my father when he had it, I'm a doctor and know what can be done so I declare and will live with dementia as a 'glorious opportunity' to help others who have only a bad picture of this disorder."[59]

Louise Morse encourages scriptural CBT.[60] This is taking the very positive messages from the New Testament, the words of Jesus and Paul, and applying them to our lives. It is like building your life on a rock solid foundation;[61] it is like protecting yourself effectively:

> *Put on all the armour that God gives, so you can defend yourself against the devil's tricks.*
>
> *Ephesians 6:11*

For Christians, including those with Alzheimer's disease, our discipline is to align our thinking with biblical truth. The default position for Christians is the word, the presence and friendship of Jesus. CBT is applying scripture to your life.

There is another more task-specific way in which CBT can be used in dementia. This is called Goal-Orientated Cognitive Rehabilitation.

---

59 Jennifer Bute; *www.gloriousopportunity.org*

60 Louise Morse; *Pathways to Hope: Spiritual insights and practical advice.* Monarch Books (2015); ISBN 978-0-85721-655-7.

61 See Matthew 7:24-27.

In this an occupational therapist or a carer will identify one or several tasks that someone with early dementia has lost the confidence or ability to do but would like to master again. They should be simple things like making a telephone call, cooking scrambled egg, writing a postcard or learning the names of your grandchildren from their photographs. There are so many possibilities.

After observing the capability of the patient, the task will be broken down into a series of steps. These will be taught a few steps at a time, on a one-to-one basis with actual participation, and repeated many times. This is quite time-consuming but has been proved to be effective. It can give back not only a practical skill but a sense of confidence and some feeling of independence.

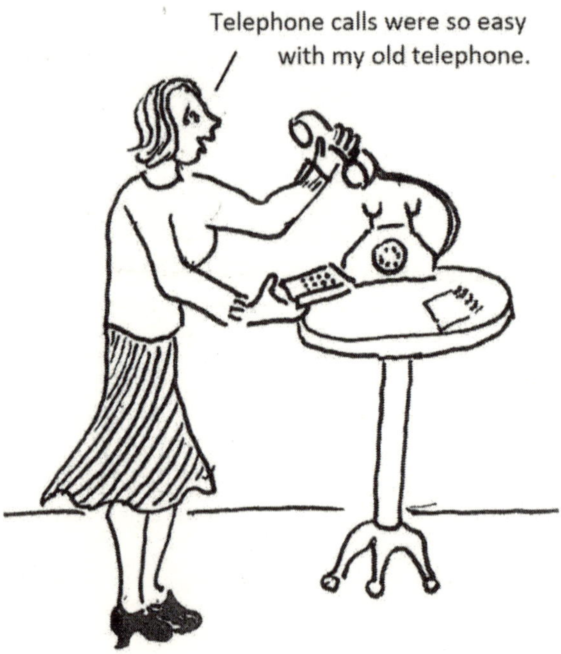

Making a telephone call.
It is a simple set of steps that can be taught.

MUSIC FOR THE BRAIN

The incredible power of music to bypass blockages in the brain has already been mentioned in the references to Sally Magnusson's powerful book.[62]

Music, especially personally meaningful music, seems able to transcend or bypass the pathologically obstructed pathways of communication. Sometimes people who have been mute for months can start singing and smiling when they hear familiar songs. As previously mentioned, Sally Magnusson's charity Playlist for Life provides helpful resources and tools to set up a playlist for this purpose.[63]

Check if you are fortunate to have a community choir in your area. Most will not demand an audition and expect you to be able to read music or be pitch-perfect! Singing together adds an important stimulation to your brain!

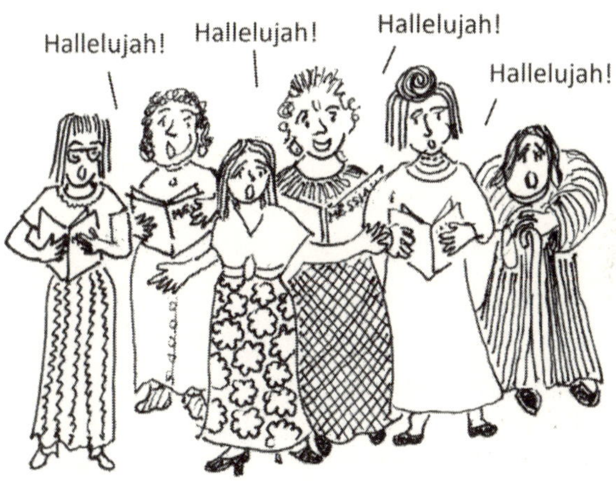

Singing together boosts brain, spirit and social contacts!

---

[62] Sally Magnusson; *Mamie. Where Memories Go – Why dementia changes everything;* Two Roads (2014).

[63] See pages 36-37 for more information.

SOCIAL INTERACTION AND MENTAL STIMULATION,

Social interaction with other people is certainly important. Tom Kitwood, in his seminal work, *Dementia Reconsidered*[64], said that "every social interaction is a neuronal event".

Building and maintaining a circle of friends and family, regular talking, discussing and even arguing is important, though the benefits of this are difficult to measure. Lonely isolation certainly makes people feel sad, afraid and they go downhill faster.

Social interaction is a form of brain stimulation and another example of the principle "use it or lose it". How you exercise your brain can be very varied, just as exercise through a tennis club may be more sociable than jogging on your own. Some people have been addicted to regular crossword puzzles and other word and number games like Sudoku for years. It is easy to encourage these devotees to continue these mind-stretching exercises on their own. To other people, these brain-games are foreign, boring or frightening. Therefore, some other people need to be drawn into exercising their minds with games in 'memory clubs', chess or bridge teams, and other regular social gatherings. The very act of getting together around a card table, a jigsaw puzzle or at a tea table with other people and a board game is a worthwhile stimulation.

Many clubs for Seniors start with a quiz. If this is played table against table, no individual need feel embarrassed. Indeed, if the range of questions is wide-ranging – history, geography, music, food, science, TV programmes, literature, transportation, current affairs, etc – some of the quietest members come up with some amazing information!

There are now electronic versions of many games and quizzes for handheld devices, but old-fashioned sources like puzzles in magazines or newspapers can be a regular worthwhile challenge.

---

[64] T. Kitwood; *Dementia Reconsidered;* Open University Press (Buckingham, UK, 1997).

Learning a new language, or brushing up on one of which you had some knowledge, is known to be good exercise for the brain. Learning to play a musical instrument is challenging, but even a simple one like a Ukulele is brain exercise. Even watching quiz programmes on the TV or other favourite shows, especially along with other people, has a role in stimulation. But personal interaction with others gives added value.

| *Remember, "Every social interaction is a neuronal event!"* |

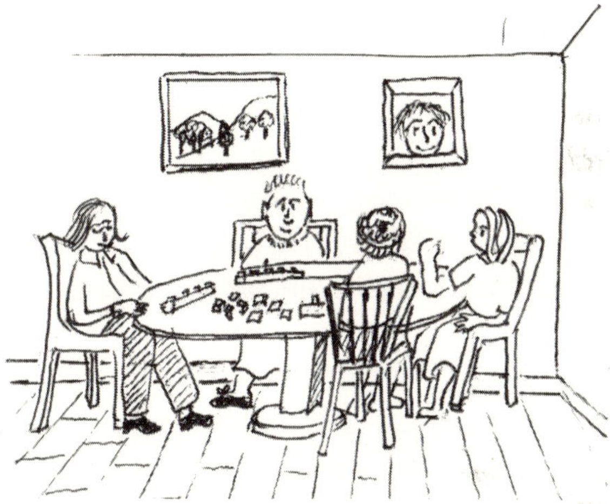

Scrabble and games keep the brain active at the memory club.

INTERGENERATION SOCIAL INTERACTION – AND FUN!

From time immemorial grandparents and grandchildren have enjoyed each other's company. In our modern divided society where large joint families are less common, it is recognised that it is mutually beneficial to deliberately bring the generations together.[65] Experience is growing with regular visits of pre-schoolers from a nursery to Seniors' day-care centres or old folks' homes. This works well, and in some places adjacent sites and facilities are planned. Joint activities include simple music,

[65] Goddard, C.; *Intergenerational care: Bringing old and young together;* Nursery Care (Feb 2017).

singing, games, storytelling, conversation, cake-decorating, picture-sharing, some exercises and, of course, laughing together. Now sociologists are trying to measure the benefits that have long been accepted as obvious!

Of course this requires leadership and supervision. There is also a need for some caution about cross-infections of not only coughs and colds, but also chicken pox – but the benefits of getting together are obvious and a joy for all.

CARING FOR PETS IS GOOD FOR HEALTH

When Dr Bill Thomas took over the running of Chase Memorial Nursing Home in New England, USA, there were 80 patients and 75% had dementia. His attempts at improving things with extra medication failed, so he planned an injection of life. He decided on shock therapy and imported two dogs, four cats and one hundred parakeets or budgerigars. After the pandemonium settled down, the patients helped to care for and feed the animals. Light was switched on in the eyes of many and some who had been mute for months started talking to the animals![66]

There is good evidence that caring for and handling animals significantly benefits health and happiness of Seniors.[67] Pets give companionship, physical contact and act as a buffer against social isolation. Love is the most important health tonic and pets are one of nature's best sources of love. Of course, with those who have dementia the benefits of pets have to be balanced against the responsibilities. A pet to care for, feed and stroke is a great motivator and even a budgie can be a good companion and is less demanding than a dog or rabbit. Sometimes simply borrowing or sharing an animal for 'pet therapy' is sensible.

---

[66] A. Gawande; *Being Mortal; Illness, Medicine and What Matters in the End;* Profile Books Ltd. (2014).

[67] Cherniack, E.P., et al.; *The Benefit of Pets and Animal-Assisted Therapy to the Health of Older Individuals;* Current Gerontology and Geriatric Research (2014); doi: 10.1155/2014/623203. Published online.

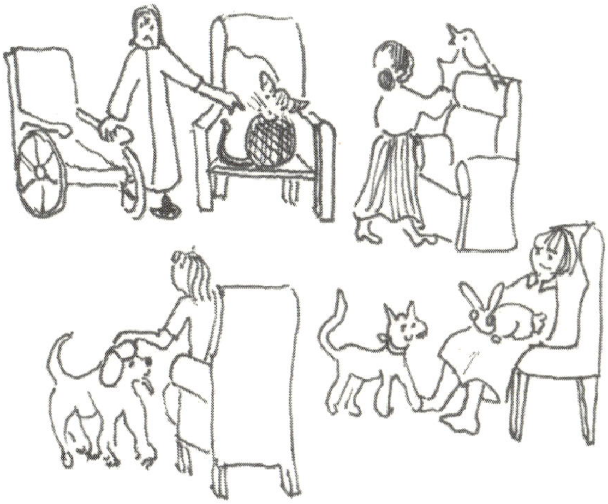

Even simple pets, budgies and goldfish can stimulate and be companions.

STRENGTHENING SPIRIT AND SOUL[68]

For many people, their religious faith is an important and integral part of who they are. For Christians, their faith gives them direction in life, strength in times of trouble, and peace when danger or uncertainty loom. The Bible contains many verses of encouragement and reasons for hope. Prayer enables believers to worship and make specific requests for help. Meeting with believing friends provides fellowship and mutual support. All these positive benefits are just what those with dementia need.

'Brain and Soul Boosting for Seniors'[69] is an effective programme developed and tested by two experienced experts, Louise Morse and Janet Jacob. It combines cognitive and spiritual stimulation with social interaction. A group with early dementia meet with a couple of leaders, about once a week, for a series of up to fifteen sessions. Each meeting has a theme, for example, Bread, Celebrations, Colours, Games, Gardens, Foods, Holidays etc. There is always a quiz, some activity, opportunities for

---

[68] See also chapter 4.
[69] L. Morse and J. Jacob; *Brain and Soul Boosting;* Pilgrims' Friend Society (London, 2016).

discussion, sharing, singing, Bible readings and prayer. The whole atmosphere is one of stimulation, fun and friendship.

CONTINUE YOUR INTEREST IN HOBBIES, HANDICRAFTS, GARDENING ETC.

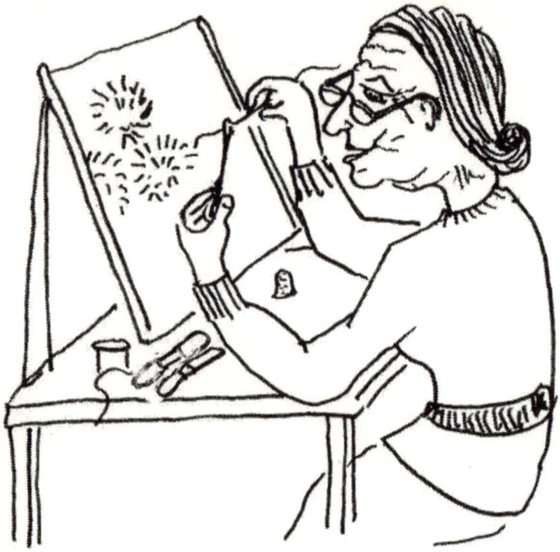

Embroidery exercises skills of eye, hand and brain.

Many, but not all, people have hobbies that have been their passion for years and are part of who they are. They probably have a vast knowledge about the subject which has been developed over years of participation and study. Obviously, some activities will not be possible in old age – hang-gliding and rally-driving come to mind! However, many hobbies can be continued into advanced years. Using the hands can stimulate the brain. Simple knitting and crocheting are very good, especially if they are with a purpose: a scarf for an old friend or squares for a charity rug. Things like drawing, painting, music or reading are good to stimulate the brain and imagination and are all to be encouraged.

KEEP UP YOUR DOMESTIC SKILLS

Most men and women have an amazing toolkit of domestic skills that they have developed and refined with years of practice. Sometimes these skills are quickly lost in a situation where everything is done for you. It is another example of "use it or lose it". Of course, some people are seriously immobile, incapable or weak, but sometimes people become weak because they stop doing things that they were able to do for themselves. Everyone appreciates having a hot meal prepared for them, either in a cafeteria or 'meals-on-wheels', but there is something satisfying about being independent and able to cope for yourself, even better if you invite a guest! This is much easier with the abundance and variety of nutritious 'ready meals' now available.

DIETARY MODIFICATIONS AND DEMENTIA

There is no evidence that taking any single item of food or any vitamin or other supplement will significantly improve any form of dementia.

However, there is growing evidence that regularly eating a 'good' mixed diet, for example a Mediterranean diet, is associated with a lower risk of dementia. If that is the case, it is likely that this will also slow the progress of dementia.

What is a Mediterranean diet? It is a diet with a high intake of cereals, fruits, fish, legumes and other vegetables. It is often rich in unsaturated fatty acids, its main source being olive oil, with a low intake of meat, poultry and saturated fatty acids. Intake of dairy products, especially yogurt and cheese, tend to be low to moderate. Meals are often accompanied by some alcohol, particularly wine. However, there is now some evidence that any alcohol is detrimental.[70]

---

[70] Topiwala A., Allan C., Valkanova V. et al.; *Moderate alcohol consumption as risk factor for adverse brain outcomes and cognitive decline: longitudinal cohort study;* BMJ2017;357:j2353.
Killian, A.; *Alcohol consumption and brain health.* Editorial. BMJ (6 Jun 2017): 357; *https://doi.org/10.1136/bmj.j2645;* BMJ 2017;357:j2645.

Vitamin D is known to be of value for older people, especially in the winter months when sunlight is in short supply. It is often given with calcium supplements to maintain bone strength. Low vitamin D concentrations have been found in those with Alzheimer's disease, but this deficiency is not the cause of the disease. The low levels probably indicate that many with dementia are undernourished, for a range of reasons. Adequate nutrition in dementia needs careful attention.

The role of medicines

There is still no medicinal cure for dementia. However, medication has a limited place in management. Although there is no cure, some drugs can relieve some symptoms for some time. Two types of medicines are used to slow the progress of Alzheimer's disease: acetylcholinesterase inhibitors (often shortened to just 'cholinesterase inhibitors' or CEIs) and NMDA receptor antagonists. The two types work in different ways.

- *The cholinesterase inhibitors.* The generic names for the CEIs are donepezil, rivastigmine and galantamine.
  This is how they are believed to work: In Alzheimer's disease there is a reduced level of acetylcholine, a chemical important in transmission of nerve impulses. The CEI drugs stop an enzyme from destroying this transmitter substance. This permits increased communication between nerve cells, so they stimulate brain activity. Unfortunately, in some people it causes insomnia and vivid dreams. This is unacceptable for some people as sleep is very important for everyone.
- The NMDA receptor antagonist is memantine. It was originally patented as Ebixa and is now also available as generic memantine. Glutamate is another chemical messenger substance between nerve cells. When brain cells are damaged by Alzheimer's disease, Glutamate is released

---

Louise Morse; *Dementia: Frank and Linda's Story;* Monarch Books (2010).

in excessive amounts, which damages more brain cells. Memantine protects brain cells by blocking the effects of excess glutamate. This is mainly recommended for those with more advanced disease or those who cannot tolerate the CEI medicines.

As we have discussed,[71] in many patients with Alzheimer's disease plaques of amyloid material have been found in and around the brain. These were believed to block nerve transmission. In the search for a cure, anti-amyloid drugs were developed and some of these, particularly Solanezumab, were used in a variety of trials. This appeared to lower brain amyloid but failed to improve cognitive function, so it failed. This emphasizes that we still do not understand the cause of the condition and there is no pharmaceutical cure on the horizon.

There are useful medicines for some conditions that make dementia worse. Examples are medications for Parkinson's disease or if the thyroid gland or the heart is not working well. These medicines must be taken regularly with a good routine and correct dosage, but they are effective for these conditions and therefore may slow or delay dementia.

Vascular dementia is the second largest group of dementia, and about 1 in 10 of those with Alzheimer's disease have a 'Mixed' type with a vascular component. Therefore, correct treatment of heart and blood vessel disease is important to limit the damage. There are powerful and effective medicines available to reduce high blood pressure and harmful cholesterol. This is part of good comprehensive care for those with dementia.

Occasionally, older patients are on so many medications that these produce symptoms of forgetfulness and drowsiness. In these patients, the stopping of many medicines result in the patient appearing to recover from dementia! Every old patient should have a check with a pharmacist or a GP at least every six months to check that they are not on too many or any inappropriate

[71] See page 49.

drugs. Do not hesitate to ask the GP, "When did this patient have his or her last medicine review?"

References

Kitwood T; *Dementia Reconsidered;* Open University Press (Buckingham, UK, 1997).

Playlist for Life
www.playlistforlife.org.uk

Dementia | Treatment summary | BNF Provided by NICE
bnf.nice.org.uk/treatment-summary/dementia.html

In Lighter Mode: Granddad's Childminding

A bright three-year-old, Jane, was just recovering from a tummy upset and Granddad had been asked to look after her while Mother went out to do some shopping. Granddad's childminding consisted of sitting in the lounge reading his newspaper while Jane played with her recent gift, a little tea set.

Jane pottered in and out and brought her Granddad several 'cups of tea' – cold water – to drink. It was a great game enjoyed by them both.

After Mum returned, Granddad told her with pride how he had been served several cups of "delicious tea", "a delightful game".

"Jane, please could you bring me one more cup of tea."

In a few moments Jane trotted down the hall into the lounge with the 'tea'. Wonderful – until Mum pointed out that the only place she could have reached for the water was the toilet bowl.

So much for Granddad's childminding!

CHAPTER SEVEN

Living with Memory Loss

Forgetfulness and the cycle of stress

Forgetfulness can be the start of dementia, and it begins like this (talking to yourself):

> "I can't remember anything."
> – Well, that's not true!
> "So, I'm not going to cope"
> – Rubbish! There are still lots of things I can do.
> "Now I'm getting stressed..."
> – Calm down and take a few deep breaths.
> "I'm stressed so I cannot concentrate, so of course I don't remember things!"

Break the cycle of stress, forgetfulness, anxiety, and depression. Do this through recognising it and reducing stress by:

- Doing things you find relaxing and enjoyable.
- Applying strategies to help you remember things.

Do some things you enjoy: gardening, listening to music, talking with a friend, walking with a dog, watching a film, taking a leisurely bath and other relaxation techniques.

Use memory strategies that suit you. If there is information you need for a forthcoming visit, repeat it out loud, write it down. Keep one little notebook of practical things to remember.

Remember names and other things by association: other people with the same name, where you were when you heard a name or a fact. Be methodical in writing down names, dates and engagements.[72]

Dr Jennifer Bute was able to keep working as a doctor for some time before she was formally diagnosed with Alzheimer's disease, by becoming very methodical about keeping her diary and her patients' notes in detail and up-to-date.[73]

Historical memory reminders

A MEMORY ALBUM OR SCRAPBOOK

This is a way to 'time travel' back through life, visit old places and look at familiar faces. With the help of family and friends, make a picture memory book, with the pictures clearly labelled and, if possible, dated.

- A series of pictures of the homes, the towns and places in which you lived and worked, major journeys you have made, the great moments that represent some main themes of your life.
- Pictures of family, childhood, brothers and sisters, children through their stages; friends of yesteryears and more recently – and get help to name and label them clearly!
  With the help of technically savvy children and grandchildren, an iPad and other tablets can be made to operate simply and effectively.
  You may have a relative who might help you record a commentary on some of your pictures – a personal voice-over about the pictures.
- Scrapbooks related to your hobbies, pastimes and work.

[72] See the section entitled 'Short-term memory joggers' on page 129.
[73] Jennifer Bute; *Dementia: A Glorious Opportunity;* Christian Medical Fellowship, Triple Helix 53:18-19 (London, 2012).

A memory box is along the same lines as the album.

Collect some small memorable keepsake items. A decorated shoebox can be a nostalgic treasure chest of items you can handle: a sports or war time medal, a lock of hair, a dried flower, a locket, a journey ticket, a sea shell, a pine cone or eucalyptus nut, an old postcard or even a valentine! Each will bring back a scene, a scent and situation that will strengthen old memories and consolidate who you are.

AUTOBIOGRAPHICAL EXERCISE

In addition to the early pictures and memorabilia, some older folk can be persuaded to chat about, dictate or write down stories from their early or middle life. Such an autobiographical exercise will help them to firm up the foundations about who they are.

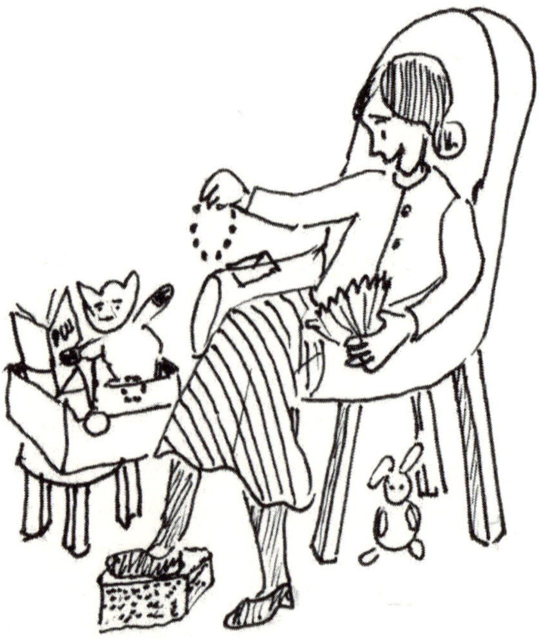

Memory box: a box of emotional rather than financial treasures!

SHORT-TERM MEMORY JOGGERS.

Use these aid memoirs as much as possible; they can limit frustrations.

Calendars and wall charts are especially important. These must have space to write family birthdays, doctor's and other appointments and even minor events, day by day. Keep the calendar near to where you sit for your meals and consult it as a routine every day.

A diary, kept carefully and used daily, or even intermittently, can have the same benefits. A few people will have the habit and discipline to use this.

Write a journal to help you remember what you have done, anyone you met and anything new, important or interesting that came up each day. Alternatively, a notebook can be used to write down important things. It is better to have just one notebook at a time. Keep these things always in the same place, along with a reliable ball-pen to write whatever comes up.

Some clocks are made to show day and date as well as time. Alarm clocks are very useful to remind you about simple things like mealtimes, when the meat in the oven should be ready, or when a visitor is due. These are now more quickly to hand with modern telephones, electronic tablets etc. and quite simple to use. (How to use the alarm on your phone or tablet could be a useful topic taught by Goal-Orientated CBT[74].)

Smartphones can be complicated, but they can be very valuable just to keep the names, numbers and addresses of family and friends. Learn a few basic things, practise looking them up and calling them. Don't worry about all the fancy things that they can do!

A noticeboard is useful. Pin on it important appointments or letters. Keep a pad of small sticky labels (Post-It labels) and a ball-pen nearby. Whenever something important comes on your

[74] See pages 112-114.

mind, write it down and and stick it up somewhere you cannot miss it.

Checklists of things to be done (and when) become really important.

Even in the 21st century, there are few things better than a little pocket notebook and a pencil or ball-pen!

Additional tools to help you

PLACES TO KEEP THINGS

Grandma said, "Have a place for everything and keep everything in its place."

- Have a simple file system for important letters and documents.
- Keep important things attached to you; glasses on a cord around your neck, keys pinned in a pocket or attached to your belt.
- Keep valuable things in one safe place, not many safe places.
- Sometimes have extras; spare pens and a second pair of glasses.
- Cupboards and drawers can be labelled with what they contain.

ROUTINES

Use a routine for your day and week; it gives your life a structure that is valuable. Update the good old pattern:

- Sunday – church
- Monday – wash day
- Tuesday – memory club
- Wednesday – exercises
- etc.

PICTURES OF PEOPLE WHO ARE IMPORTANT TO YOU

One of the first things people find difficult to remember is people and their names. With mobile telephone cameras, it is now much easier to take a quick picture and keep a record of people. (This is another skill that can be taught by Goal-Orientated CBT[75].)

If you cannot manage the camera phone yourself, many younger carers have this skill and will be proud to do this for you. Ask them to photograph all visitors. Label the pictures boldly and add birthdays.

A DAILY DIARY MEMORY-BOOSTING REGIME

Sleep is important in clearing the brain.[76] Recalling and reviewing things before you sleep has been known to stick them in your memory. It is an effective method that has been used by students over the years.

Some people with early memory loss have used this. Near the end of the day, write down in a notebook or diary the main events of the day and the people you met. It should be a short, factual list in your own hand and words. As you sleep, these details have a better chance of fixing.

Note: It is not a literary exercise; you are not emulating Samuel Pepys!

The next evening, review yesterday's activities and people before you record today's. At the weekend, review the events of the week and refresh your memory of names and events in this simple, useful way.

---

[75] See pages 112-114.

[76] See page 186.

In Lighter Mode: Bad Memory

A good thing about having a bad memory:
that way a joke can be funny every time you hear it!

A clear conscience is a certain sign of having only a short-term memory.

The secret of happiness is a good sense of humour and a bad memory!

- My memory is so bad.
- How bad is it?
- How bad is what?

My memory is so bad. That's why every party I organise turns out to be a 'surprise party'!

Don't worry, I never hold grudges, because I have a deliberately bad memory.

Two good things about having Alzheimer's disease:

1. You can wrap up your own Christmas presents and they will still be a surprise.
2. You are meeting new friends every day.

I'm not speeding, Officer, but I have to get there quickly or I will forget where I'm going.

Everything is new – "Been there, done that, forgotten the lot, so going again will be a completely fresh experience!"

I took this course – "Breakthrough in memory loss" – but I still can't remember why I agreed to marry him!

One excellent thing about being over 60:
we did most stupid things before the
social media exposed them to everybody!

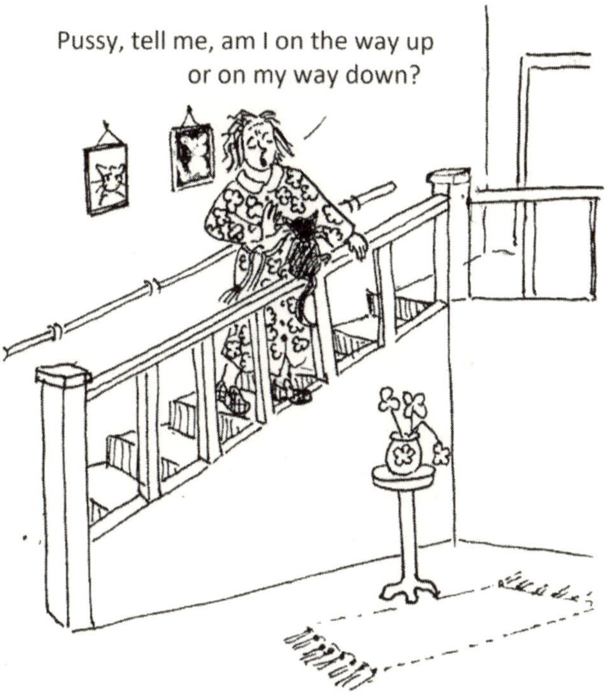
Pussy, tell me, am I on the way up
or on my way down?

Asking for directions.

CHAPTER EIGHT

Practical Strategies for the Major Symptoms

Not everyone will want to read the next few pages, but they contain really useful advice for anyone who has family or a friend with advanced dementia. The information is invaluable for all carers.

We will also look at examples from the life of Fred, who has Alzheimer's, and his wife Mary.

Carers: two vital matters

Be bold and persistent to ask for all the medical and social support possible.

Look after your own physical, mental, social and spiritual needs and health. The wellbeing of the one you care for will depend on your health. Take care.[77]

Create a relaxing environment

Keep rooms simple and tidy, get rid of confusing clutter and label things with big labels. Plenty of light is good, but only gentle light at night. Make sure that the toilet is obvious and minimise reflections and mirrors that can cause confusion.

[77] See chapter 10.

Create a den with favourite books and furnishing, and make the place smell nice, for example with lavender perfume.

Touch is an important sense and, where appropriate, hugs, hand-holding and massaging are helpful. Stroking soft toys can help some people.

Petting pets is useful; encourage dogs, cats, even fish in a tank.

Some people with progressing dementia feel restless and still have considerable strength. Walking, either with others or with a dog, can use their energy and help them to relax.

Fred had always been fond of dogs, but felt that when he was working he could not give the time to give it walks. When he retired, or actually was made redundant, his son gave him a dog – "Now you have the time and you will both enjoy the exercise." Toby was a great companion when the Alzheimer's set in. He knew the routes and for several years the dog walked the man and brought him safely home. Toby did not object to the oft repeated stroking that was one of Fred's repetitive mannerisms. Toby always stayed calm when glasses or keys went missing!

Aggression, agitation or anxiety

AGGRESSION

Verbal aggression, shouting, or physical aggression, throwing or pushing may occur. Sometimes it is sudden, with no apparent reason, or sometimes it follows a frustration.

Aggression doesn't always happen, and sometimes is only for a phase, but it is horrible and requires help and support. Carers, remember, it is not your fault. Try not to identify with the details but rather the feelings behind the words. Try to find a cause; is the person in pain or discomfort? Avoid possible triggers. It may often be due to misinterpreting what the person thinks is happening to them. It may be associated with anxiety, or misunderstanding what you are trying to do to help them, for example, to undress them in the toilet. Fear may be the issue because the person does not recognise you, or anger at not being able to make a machine work. The aggression may be associated with hallucinations or delusions.

Interventions include shifting the focus to some other activity or just leaving the room. Protect yourself from emotional or physical bashing. Ask for help and support if it recurs. Avoid unnecessary stress and keep to a simple routine. Make life less boring, look at memory books or take a walk. Use calming words, touch or music. Singing along can be therapeutic.

Fred used to get upset and aggressive if he could not work the remote buttons for the TV. He had always been good with technology! Mary could usually manage it, but she had a great formula for settling Fred. For years he had been in charge of the sound and lighting for the Christmas Nativity play in the church. Mary had a great CD of the music and carols, and it worked a treat, especially when she and Fred sang along! The children's voices and the message of peace and goodwill was a tonic that restored calm in agitated moments, even in the height of summer!

AGITATION OR ANXIETY

These usually occur when the person is feeling frustrated and distressed. A partner will often know the triggers, the things that set this off, but it is always distressing.

Forgetfulness and losing things like glasses causes distress. Listen to the frustration. If the cause of symptoms could be something physical, discuss it with the GP.

- Avoid triggers, and use and repeat calming phrases and reassurance as distraction.
- Keep spare glasses, ball pens etc. if these are often 'lost'.
- Distractions are valuable, for example, a car ride or purposeful exercise (walking or swimming help and burn energy).
- A safe and relaxing environment is good and gentle and appropriate touching and holding hands is comforting.
- The right music is such good therapy. It should be on the NHS!

- Life-story work is very worthwhile. Get them to tell you about what was important in their lives. Make a scrapbook of stories and pictures. See *www.caringmemories.net* to make an electronic memory book.

Fred and Mary's grandson Josh was a bright 12-year-old who used to come in at the weekend. He was interested in computers and aeroplanes. When he heard that Fred did his military service in the RAF, he used to ask him about his time in Cyprus, servicing the planes. Then he scanned pictures of Fred in uniform and some of the planes he knew and made an album. Soon other members of the family started asking Fred about his early years and it became a family project and a real *aide-memoire*.

Confusion or depression

CONFUSION

The person may not recognize familiar people, places or things, may forget relationships, call family members by other names or become confused as to where home is. They may also forget the purpose of common items, such as a pen or a fork.

- Stay calm and try not to take offence if you are not recognised or are called a wrong name.
- Give brief simple explanations, not lengthy statements.
- Use memory books and photographs to remind about important people and demonstrate how to use objects without making an issue of things.

DEPRESSION

Depression can come on top of dementia.

The carer may notice that the person has lost interest, is withdrawn, feels sad and tired, and either sleeps too much or cannot sleep.

- Medication is often worthwhile for depression.
- The distraction strategies suggested above are all useful: animals, outings, old photos and DVDs, and exercise in the company of others.
- Multisensory therapy helps some: music, coloured lights, smells and touch all at the same time.
- Sometimes it is possible to give positive validation about a particular issue. If the person is crying for her mother who died 50 years ago, don't deny the loss she feels, but say something comforting: "Your mum was lovely. What did she used to cook for birthdays?"
- Companionship and laughter can be magic.

For several years, Mary used to take Fred to the 'memory café' each week. There, several of the folk used to share their stories about the mix-ups they had caused. It was a good time of companionship and laughter. Also, Mary met several other carers who were struggling as she was.

Repetition

A person with Alzheimer's may do or say something over and over again – a word, a question or activity, probably looking for comfort, security or some familiarity. They may also pace about or undo a recently completed task. These actions can be stressful for others.

- Stay calm, be patient, reassure the person with a friendly voice and gentle touch.
- Learn to expect and not be irritated by repetition.
- Provide a simple answer that seems to satisfy. When the question is repeated, do not be afraid to repeat the same reassuring answer.
- Look for a reason behind the repetition and try to find a specific cause. Rather than react to what the person is saying or doing, focus on the emotion; think about how they are feeling.

- Turn the action into an activity. If they are moving their hand up and down the table, provide a cloth and suggest they do some polishing.
- When you have found an answer to a repeated question that calms and satisfies, do not be afraid to use it repeatedly.

Suspicion or hallucinations

SUSPICION

Memory loss and confusion may cause things to be perceived in new, unusual ways. Individuals may become suspicious or accuse others of theft or improper behaviour. The person may misinterpret what they see and hear.

- Don't take offence. Allow the individual to express ideas.
- Listen to what is troubling them and try to understand. Acknowledge his or her opinions.
- Be reassuring and let the person know you care and take them seriously.
- Don't argue or try to convince; just offer a simple answer.
- Don't overwhelm the person with explanations or reasons.
- Switch the focus and engage the individual in an activity, or ask for help with a task: "Let us make a cup of tea," or, "Let us look at this photo album together."
- Duplicate any lost items if the person is often searching for a specific item: a ballpoint pen, glasses, hairbrush etc.

HALLUCINATIONS

A *misinterpretation* is trying to pick up a leaf from the floral pattern in the carpet, or seeing your reflection and thinking it's a stranger.

Most distressing is not recognising your 'nearest and dearest'.

Fred asked the visiting nurse, "Who is that old lady who hangs around the house?" Gently she asked him, "What is your wife like?" He smiled and described the lovely young woman who was kind and the mother of his children!

A *hallucination* is different; it is seeing, hearing, smelling or even feeling things that are not there at all. They may be part of dementia, but medications and infections can also cause them. They can be horrible and cause suspicion and fear, but they may also give an insight into the type of dementia. Tell the medical team about them.

- Don't argue about them or deny them; that cannot make them go away and will cause distress.
- Make sure it is not a misinterpretation; check the lights or reflections.
- Keep a diary to see if there is a repeating pattern or a trigger event.
- If it is horrible, give comfort and reassurance as if it were real. For example, if the person is afraid of a bird hallucination, give a cuddle and say, "I will chase it away." That is not a lie; you can make it go away. Distraction is sometimes appropriate. If carers stick to a routine response, the upset declines.
- Check if the person is getting enough food, drink and sleep and that the hallucination is not a side-effect of medicines. Sometimes you may need a reality check.

Fred's friend Mavis at the 'memory café' used to say, "Oh, don't worry about me; Basil keeps me company. He comes around for afternoon tea." Mary knew Mavis had Parkinson's and hallucinations and thought that Basil was imaginary so she told her nurse about this. The next day, the nurse was with Mavis at teatime and on the windowsill was Basil, the squirrel!

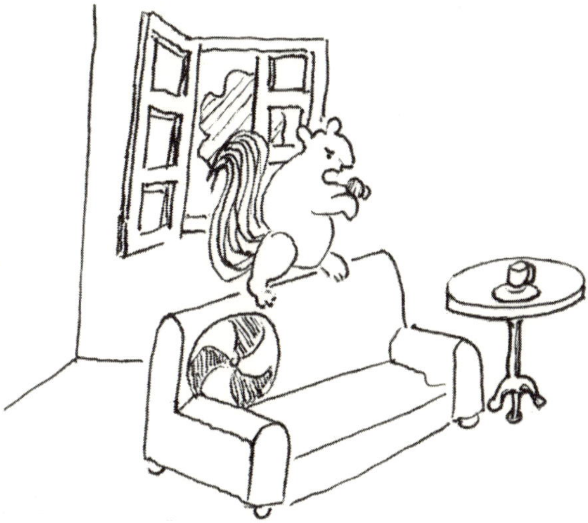

Basil the squirrel came for tea!

Sleeplessness

Sleep deprivation is a form of torture. People with dementia often sleep lightly. Also remember, a sleep-deprived carer cannot do his or her tough job properly!

Getting people to bed and asleep for as much of the night as possible is so important.

- Exercise tires the body in preparation for sleep.
- Daytime napping, often from boredom, can lead to night-time insomnia. Socialising, activities and getting out and about decrease daytime napping.
- Seek help to keep people busy during the day.
- Check medication: Donepizil increases insomnia in some people.
- Have a regular bedtime routine. Use the recognised household pattern: warm drink, TV off, possibly soft music, pyjamas or nightdress on, toileting, warm bed, affectionate "good night", and some like a short prayer:

Now I lay me down to sleep,
I pray the Lord, my soul to keep.
Guard me, Jesus, through the night
and wake me with the morning light.
Amen.

Lord, make me joyful in hope,
patient in trouble and faithful in prayer.[78] Amen.

- Put away daytime things, especially clothes, so that a confused person will not arise in the night and put on their clothes. Some care homes give night staff dressing gowns to wear over uniforms and get them to speak quietly: "Shush, time for sleep."
- Think of appropriate lighting: a small light to give reassurance and possibly bathroom light that comes on triggered by an infrared beam. Ideally, a person with dementia should be able to see the toilet commode from the bed and the bed from the toilet. Variations on this are possible.
- A warm bed in a cool room encourages staying in bed!
- Medical conditions, aches and pains, constipation and urinary infections cause discomfort and wakefulness. Check these things and try simple painkillers. Medication and sleeping pills were common and still have a limited place under careful supervision. (A dose giving a daytime hangover and napping is no good though.) An alcoholic 'nightcap' was also recommended by some, but recent evidence indicates that even small daily doses of wine or sherry can cause liver damage.
- Night-time snacks help some with insomnia. They are useful if pre-wrapped and ready so as to cause little disturbance.

[78] Based on Romans 12:12.

Walking about or wandering

Walking about in an aimless manner, indoors or outside, is quite common in people with dementia. It is worrying that they may do themselves some harm and a nightmare if they go missing. When the 'lost person' returns or is found, the risk is that carers are so relieved and angry that they lock all doors and watch every movement that so that the poor 'culprit' feels like a prisoner.

Solutions to wandering are based on possible causes, for example, pain, need for the toilet but no awareness of what to do, feeling trapped, wanting to go 'home', boredom, anxiousness and stress, confusion, thinking that they should be doing something.

Hyperactivity may be a phase of the dementia. They may find the repeated movement comforting.

In fact the cause may be a combination of these things.

- First check for physical problems or medication that could be the cause and may be changed.
- Use any of the strategies given earlier in this chapter,[79] to counter boredom or frustration and give calm and pleasant sensations.
- Exercise, again, is important. Find folk willing to walk with them, and in some towns there are 'walky talky' clubs for groups of older folk.
- If someone is trying to leave, better not to restrain or argue. Get on the right clothes, go with them, then distract, relax and return home. But it takes much time and patience!
- If walking outdoors is impossible, distract with the life story book, music or dancing on the spot to burn up energy. If the person is a determined walker, perhaps try, "Why not sit down for a while; we don't want you to conk out!"

---

[79] For example, see page 139.

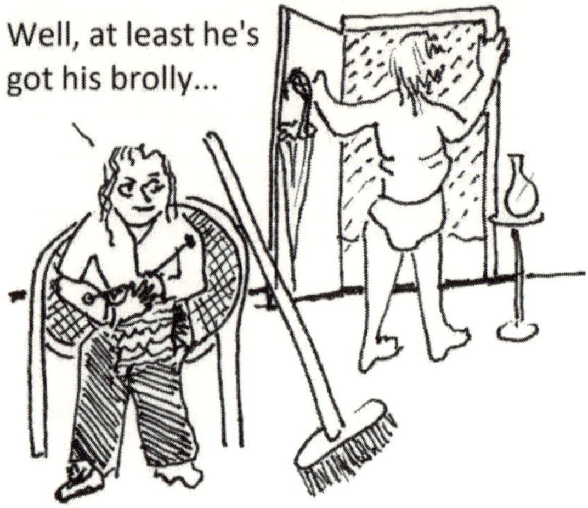

"There he goes again, escaping, inadequately dressed.
At least he's got his brolly."

Unwanted exiting from the house can be a nightmare. Locks may be necessary but can be a hazard. Big 'DON'T USE THIS DOOR' signs or painting the door to make it less obvious can help.

Despite best efforts, loved ones get lost. Keep identification cards in pockets; identification bracelets and tracking devices can be useful. Some 'wanderers' have usual haunts to which they go. Speak to the staff at these places, and sometimes local friends and businesses can act as a 'neighbourhood watch'.

If a person gets lost, have a recent photo, description of clothes and information about where they worked, lived and hobbies. When the lost is found, relax – no harm was done; it was not your fault – but talk to everyone who can help: family, GP, neighbours etc.

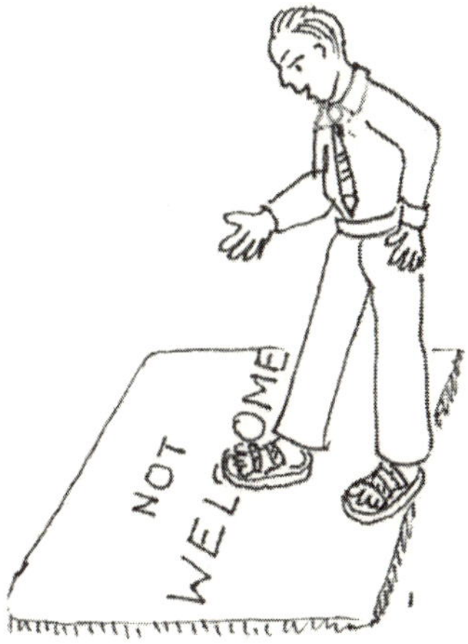

Bold signs can discourage worrying 'wandering' away from home.

Personal care in later stages of dementia

Every person with dementia will have a different pattern of illness, symptoms and rate of progress. In the end, dementia can be a fatal disease because nearly all bodily functions depend on the brain, including breathing and circulation. Some with dementia die from other conditions as the body becomes frail, immobile and defences fail. Others end up as vulnerable as newborn infants, do not know who they are, cannot recognise their nearest and dearest, cannot walk, talk, feed themselves or control their bowels. Each and every symptom requires and deserves professional and loving care.

A friend who was the personal carer for his wife at home, right up to her last breath, has shared some of his detailed experience. He described some of the things he found most useful during the last stages of care. They are included in the list below.

- *Services and equipment*
  Contact and access the Local Authority Social Services through your General Practitioner or family doctor. For his wife they provided an excellent carer, at first for 12 hours a week, but later for 32. Without this carer and family

support, he would not have been able to give what amounted to the rest of the 24-hour care! Payment for carers will vary in different places and circumstances, and requires negotiation.

The Local Authority Social Work Service were very helpful in providing and loaning practical equipment. After mobility was difficult, this included a special bed and a hoist for toileting, a battery-operated bath lift, a commode and an external ramp for the wheelchair.

Special Services were made available and were very helpful: Continence Support, Dietetic Support and Occupational Therapy.

Purchase of a riser and recliner chair was valuable at one stage when strength to sit or stand up was failing.

- *Social contact, practical skills and brain stimulation*

  Visits from family and friends are important. Sometimes church friends come to pray with the person and family. Many people find visiting someone with dementia is challenging because they are embarrassed that they cannot talk naturally; the conversation seems one-sided if the patient is silent, repeat themselves or refer to distant past events.[80]

  Using a range of simple manual skills at the appropriate stage gives satisfaction to many patients. These include simple knitting squares, doing easy jigsaw puzzles, colouring children's books, lacing up cards with holes punched in them, and underlining or highlighting books, even if they cannot read and understand them.

  Music is of special value to those with dementia. It has the power to transport the mind back to happy times and places. My friend used to play piano pieces and hymns that he and his wife loved. The charity Playlist for Life helps

[80] See page 102 for helpful advice on visiting someone with dementia.

and encourages families to make a personal collection of favourite music.[81]

Being read to can bring contentment. Familiar books, favourite Bible passages, poems and rhymes or children's stories are useful.

Selected recorded books suit some people.

Special interests can be stimulated, for example, a bird feeder or bird table placed just outside the bedroom window, or a small fish tank. These can be a delight to those interested in birds, fish and nature.

- *Safety and nourishment*

  Escaping from the house or even opening the door of a moving car can be a problem. Careful locking up and using 'child locks' on passenger doors is important.

  Aspects of eating can be a problem. Finger foods are good when holding cutlery becomes difficult. Pouching, holding food in the mouth and reluctance or difficulty swallowing can be an issue. Liquidising food may be necessary. Feeding can be very slow and requires time and patience. Inadequate nutrient intake can be a problem, but supplements like 'Complan' and extra cream with puddings and drinks can boost intake. A record of regular weights gives a useful indication about the nutrition of patients.

References

Morse, Louise; *Dementia: Frank and Linda's Story;* Monarch Books (Oxford, 2010)

Andrews, June and House, Allan; *10 Helpful Hints for Carers who live with people with dementia;* University of Stirling (2009)

Bute, Jennifer; *Dementia, Glorious Opportunity; www.gloriousopportunity.org*

[81] See pages 36-37.

In Lighter Mode: Seniors' Brain Exercise

Cover the answer until you have made up your own mind. Relax and begin.

1. Johnny's mother had three children. The first child was named April, the second child was named May. What was the third child's name?

   Answer: Johnny, of course.

2. The assistant in the butcher shop is five feet ten inches tall, and his shoe size is 13. What does he weigh?

   Answer: Meat.

3. Before Mt. Everest was discovered, what was the highest mountain in the world?

   Answer: Mt. Everest; it just wasn't discovered yet.

4. What word in the English Language is always spelled incorrectly?

   Answer: Incorrectly.

5. How much earth is there in a hole that measures two feet by three feet by four feet?

    Answer: None. There is no earth in a hole.

6. Billy was born on December 28th, yet his birthday is always in the summer. How is this possible?

    Answer: Billy lives in Australia.

7. In California you cannot take a picture of a man with a wooden leg. Why not?

    Answer: You can't take pictures with a wooden leg. You need a camera or a smartphone to take pictures.

8. If you were running a race, and you passed the person in 2nd place, what place would you be in now?

    Answer: You would be in 2nd. Well, you passed the person in 2nd place, not 1st.

9. Which is correct to say: "The yolk of the egg are white" or "The yolk of the egg is white"?

    Answer: Neither, the yolk of the egg is yellow.

10. Without using a calculator:

    You are driving a bus from London to Milford Haven in Wales.
    In London 17 people get on the bus.
    In Reading 6 people get off the bus and 9 people get on.
    In Swindon, 2 people get off and 4 get on.

In Cardiff, 11 people get off and 16 people get on.
In Swansea, 3 people get off and 5 people get on.
You then arrive at Milford Haven.
Question. Without looking back on the previous page, how old is the bus driver?

> Answer: Oh, for goodness sake! Don't you remember your own age? It was you driving the bus! [82]

Don't worry – 95% of people fail most of the questions! You do not really have brain failure; you may have attention deficit and a lack common sense!

---

[82] From Dr Andrew Young and others.

CHAPTER NINE

'Comfortable Dementia' – The SPECAL Method of Care

This is a whole method of managing early dementia.

SPECAL stands for 'SPecialised Early Care for ALzheimer's disease'. The emphasis is to try to understand how individual people with dementia see the world, and then fit care for them into their individual view of who they are. Such specific targeted care makes life more comfortable and less confusing for those whose memories have some big gaps about recent events, though they may have clear remembrance of important things from their past. Often they feel they are still living in past years and situations.

The system has shown a range of real benefits. It increases the person's confidence and slows the rate of deterioration. Also it reduces the need for medication, enables the person to remain in their own home for significantly longer and minimises the distress of moving to a care home or other facility. These benefits are not only for the person with dementia, but also for their family and their carers.

To use the method fully requires detailed training and much time, patience and continuity of care. Most carers looking after those with dementia do not have the training or time, but the method contains many important insights into how people with dementia see the world.

Carers who do not have the time or opportunity to apply the whole method can apply some of the principles and elements when helping any patients with dementia.

The whole technique was developed by Peggy Garner while looking after her mother-in-law, and was described in detail by Oliver James in his award-winning book *Contented Dementia.* [83]

In the introduction James states that "however advanced the illness, the real person who means so much to you is still there, ... a great deal of the mind and the emotional self of the person with dementia is still functioning."

Or as Louise Morse puts it, "you may lose your brain, but you cannot lose your soul"!

The method was carefully assessed and commended by the Alzheimer's Society, the Royal College of Nursing and Dr Jennifer Bute.

Because the method is well acclaimed and has been useful to many, a whole chapter is used to summarize the book. This gives a good picture of the technique with numerous personal examples.

The memory and the photo album

The helpful illustration of memory in dementia as a photograph album from which a number of pictures, especially more recent ones, are missing, was described earlier.[84] The 'older pictures' appear more real and dementia sufferers feel they are living in that world. Unfortunately, the world has moved on but you have to try to make sense of it from the older pictures. It is frightening because you don't recognise many of the people around you. Indeed, sometimes you do not know who you are yourself, and that is terrifying.

Penny prefers to refer to people with Alzheimer's disease or dementia not as patients, but rather "clients". This sounds less frightening because they do require special care, even if they are

---

[83] Oliver James; *Contented Dementia?;* Vermilion, Ebony Publishing (2009).
[84] See page 127.

close relatives and loved ones. I will use the term clients in my account, but prefer to remember that every person is a cherished loved one to close friends and relatives.

Because dementia affects each individual's brain in a slightly different way, and because each person's memory will be specific to their own earlier life, how you can help a person will depend on these two variable factors. The dementia client's earlier memories are needed to provide a bridge and interpret something of what is going on in their brains today.

The SPECAL method

The whole SPECAL method of helping those with dementia requires a lot of time and attention to detail. It is very well set out in Oliver James' book and this should be studied by anyone who is the primary carer for someone with the condition. Diligently and carefully applied, it can bring comfort to the client, their families and carers during an extended period of the illness.

Here is just a taster of the main components of SPECAL. It is valuable for anyone wanting to understand about dementia as it explains some of the most common features of behaviour and how to deal with them. For the detail, you should read the book.

The SPECAL method of helping depends on learning from the individual:

- What they can clearly remember, usually from their early life.
- What interests them: hobbies, family, gardening, cooking, TV, their job or profession, sports, etc.

They alone know what these things are, and you have to find them out.

This becomes the Primary Theme of their lives to which you refer back.

Finding out about this is difficult because of the three cardinal rules of the SPECAL method:

- Do not ask questions. You must not worry them by asking questions, particularly about recent events which they cannot clearly remember.
- Agree with everything that the person says.
- Do not contradict or correct, but rather endorse them.

These basic principles are difficult and counterintuitive for people in the health professions as they often start by asking questions about symptoms. The principles are also difficult for those committed to absolute truth-telling. We need to learn how to respond to the real world as seen by those with severe dementia. This is often the world of old pictures in their photo album rather than what is going on in the world around them.

QUESTIONS

Sometimes even simple questions cannot be understood by clients, and the inability to answer them is frightening. He or she thinks, "I cannot even answer a simple question, I must have a dreadful disease." Questions are toxic to people with dementia. But you need to know details of their background to help them effectively. Careful listening is vital.

Communication is an important aspect of life, and this is also true for those with dementia. If you start with direct questions, this can cause emotional distress and a client will clam up. An opening gambit using the word 'we' is valuable, for example, "I wonder if we should..." or, "It might be a good idea if we..." (do something). Rather than a question, these non-threatening introductions can initiate conversation.

As dementia progresses, simple conversation becomes more difficult, repetition lapsing into dreary silence. To break out of this, Penny Garner in her SPECAL method recommends Verbal Ping-Pong, a conversation game. This can activate their interest in their favourite topics and improve their sense of well-being. First, think of the client's favourite subjects of conversation: perhaps a hobby or a story from long ago. This is your ball. After some initial bumbling phrases, getting 'warmed up', you can knock a few balls across. Perhaps it might be about a pet dog, if that is a favourite topic. Listen carefully to the response and try to keep it going in a gentle, non-threatening manner with the client's special interests in view. Some statements may be nonsensical, but if it gives a feeling of comfortable communication, this is worthwhile. It takes careful concentration and repeated words of praise to keep the game going, but it can revitalise your interaction with the client.

Repetition is a feature of dementia, especially repeated questions. This is the result of limited short-term memory and consequent anxiety. To deal with this, Penny Garner recommends a method she calls Spotting. This is identifying and listing the commonest questions, and then listing and testing out the most satisfactory and reassuring answers. Start with what you think will be the best answer, and then others, until you discern what is the most positive response from the client. Penny is keen on carers making lists of questions that the clients ask and lists of possible responses. Once found, a good response can be repeated every time the question is asked, because the client will have forgotten it. You should also share this information with others who also care for the client.

Obviously, some questions are difficult to respond to. "Where is my husband Jack? He hasn't been to see me for ages." That may be a natural question when he has been dead for five years, but giving the lady the bald fact will cause her a shock and a bitter pang of grief. Then, if she asks the same question an hour later because she has forgotten and you repeat the sad news, she will have another period of anguish and grief. It is important to find a response that is understandable and will leave her with a positive feeling. "Jack isn't around at present. You know how busy he was and you know he always loves you!"

NEVER CONTRADICT, RATHER AFFIRM

The feelings of those with dementia are important and fragile because of the anxiety from not remembering things. Penny Garner suggests a simple classification for our feelings as *Green* (normal, comfortable and confident feelings), *Red* (deep trauma, anxiety and even terror), and *Amber* (an intermediate state). In normal life, if there are causes for anxiety we have ways of dealing with our feelings. In dementia, when your sense of autonomy and authority is threatened, feelings go quickly to RED: alert, panic and distress. A client's feelings must be calmed through a stage of *Amber* to *Green* (peaceful confidence).

Keeping the feelings of clients in the areas of *Green,* wellbeing, is a major objective. This is why it is important to affirm, endorse and even associate yourself with a client's unlikely statements. This is powerful. If they enjoy recycling, retelling old familiar stories, even if they are partly fictitious, this is to be welcomed, even encouraged. By retelling, a client will feel comfortable, "in the *Green* zone".

THE PRIMARY THEME

When helping and caring for someone who has progressive problems with memory, especially memory of recent events, where 'many recent photos are missing from their album', it is useful to have a Primary Theme. This is the SPECAL term for a strong picture and situation from the past in which the person feels comfortable, confident, valued. This could be the time when they were the hub of family life or running a business, or captain of a sports club, or chairing a charity committee or just deeply devoted to a hobby like gardening. From this past *Green* era, this situation of strength, they are helped through the frightening uncertainties of their present situation.

To identify the Primary Theme for a client may appear obvious from their life history, special interests, enthusiasms, achievements and hobbies. However, it sometimes requires the detective work of Sherlock Holmes and the psychoanalysis of

Sigmund Freud. Seek what they feel is their 'finest hour', something they are happy about and easily talk about. They should have some strong long-term and warm, *Green* memory pictures. They should feel a sense of ownership and expertise about the theme. Choose carefully regarding Primary Theme, and test things out before concluding.

To strengthen the recall and impact of the *Green* Primary Theme, try to find a phrase, a gesture and an object. For example, Robert had always been keen on flying and his years in the RAF were the happiest of his life. Subsequently, he became very interested in the flight and identification of birds.

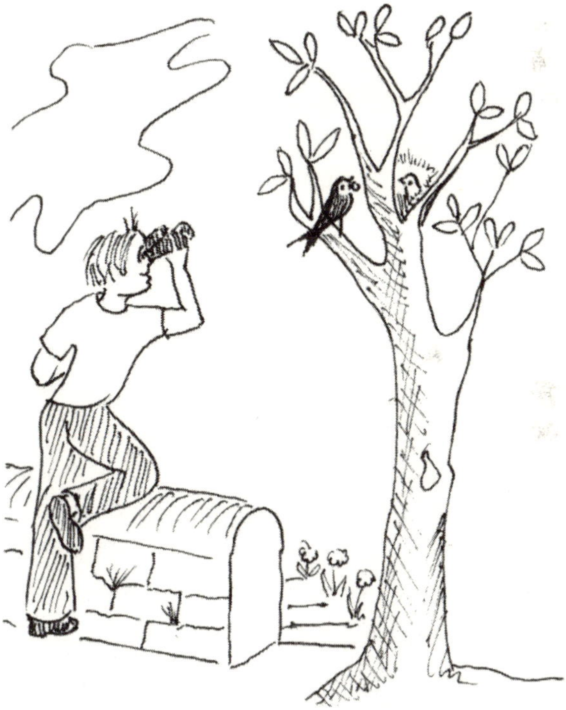

Robert, ex-RAF was always looking out for aeroplanes and birds.

A pair of binoculars were a prop that immediately took Rob back to their use in identifying either aeroplanes or birds. Later, when his memory for many things had gone, you only had to hold up your clenched hands in front of your eyes as if they were "binocs" and say, "Check what's flying in!" and he smiled broadly, instantly transported back to his *Green* time in the RAF.

Share the information about the Primary Theme with the whole team who look after the client. With the words, objects and gestures, this can transport the client back to that situation of comfort and confidence and increase the prospect of 'wrap-around 24-hour care' wherever the client is staying.

THE HEALTH THEME

The Primary Theme is to give the clients a sense of their own independence, capability and wellbeing. Without losing this, another theme from the 'old photos' is called the Health Theme. This will help the client with daily activities like eating, toileting, dressing and even accepting help. The purpose is to find an acceptable reason to take advice and suggestions. The Health Theme is based on being sensible, doing things to maintain health and avoid illness, and those with early dementia can accept this.

Review the earlier years 'pictures' for illnesses that required some actions, therapy or medication to get life back on track, for example, an earlier back problem that required rest and sensible exercise, or a bowel problem that required care about regular eating, sensible diet and 'prompt response to nature's call'. The Health Theme can be used for practical matters: "We need to get our feet up regularly to take the weight off our sore hips," or, "We must eat a regular nutritious diet to keep up our health."

Visits to doctors or practice nurses can be traumatic. These professions are trained to ask leading questions, not realising how toxic this can be for people who are already anxious about their memories. Always try to see, and prime, the medical interviewer beforehand with a written or a spoken message about the client's condition and any specific problem. Forewarn the client: "We need to see the doctor to get checked over. It is sensible to look after our health." Many clients will recognise a sense of ownership for "my medical needs". After the visit, the recommendation of a health professional can be useful: "The doctor says we must try to get out for a walk every day."

EXPLAINING THINGS

"What is going on?"

When a client cannot understand what is happening, he gets anxious, and his feelings shift to *Amber* and even *Red.* They cannot work out the comings and goings of family, carers and others. Therefore *never* leave the room, either for a moment or for a longer period, without explaining to the client that you are going, and why. You really need two explanations: one, that you are leaving, and second, the reason for going.

Explaining departures must be modified with the client and circumstances. Often, simple reasons to do with personal care are quite acceptable: "I'm off to the loo," or some other appropriate toilet phrase. It is probably better not to say, "I'm going to make a phone call," because then the client may wonder, "What is he telephoning about, and why?"

Starting your explanation with the phrase "I'm going" may cause a moment of fear ("I'm being deserted.") Unexplained departure of the carer can make a client feel insecure and provoke alarm.

As you did for the Primary Theme, you may need to test out some alternative explanations to find one that the client understands, is satisfied with and feels no need for further enquiries. Some explanations get the endorsement of the client. One husband used to say, "I need to smarten up," and his wife gave permission for departure with the phrase, "Good idea! You look a right mess." Another husband found it necessary to read in the toilet. He signalled his departure by picking up the paper and tucking it under his arm and his wife would say, "I know where you are going!"

Absence explanations are also important, especially when the main carer has to leave a client with a deputy or substitute carer.

An explanation that is seen as useful or understandable to the client is best: "I'm off to get in food supplies," or, "I need to pick up the grandchildren," or "I'm going through to the computer to check e-mails and see if there is any news from the family." Again, it is good to list alternatives, try them out and choose whatever leaves the client comfortable.

Explain the introduction and presence of a substitute carer. As the condition progresses, more help will be needed. Return to the Primary Theme and when a substitute comes to help, it is useful at first for her or him to come enquiring about some question regarding the Primary Theme. For example, when Robert, who was a keen birdwatcher, needed extra help, Janice joined. She started her first session by asking him, "What exactly is the difference between a swallow and a swift?" Delighted to be able to expound a favourite topic, Janice was accepted without being noticed as a substitute carer!

THE ALTRUISTIC TRIGGER, AS A BRAKE IN DANGEROUS SITUATIONS

Sometimes a client sets off to do something that is dangerous and should be stopped for safety's sake. Car keys in hand, Sam was walking out of the door stating that he *must* drive down to his old shop where he is needed. Explanations based on his Primary or Health themes could not stop him. He was determined. However, Sam was devoted to his grandson Pete, who had severe diabetes and needed frequent insulin. "Sam, you know that insulin is essential for young Pete. His mum needs the car this afternoon to go and collect supplies of insulin which are life-saving for the boy. A bit of trouble at the shop will settle. We must make Pete's life top priority today." Sam immediately recognised what the car should be used for. Pete was priority.

Penny believes there should be an emergency Altruistic Trigger for all clients, but this may be hard to identify. Moreover, some criticise this strategy as sometimes using blatant deceit to make someone who has impaired cognisance act in a particular way, even if it is in the way of safety and comfort. The alternative in some cases would be strong physical or pharmacological constraint which could be much more damaging to someone struggling to keep a hold on some sort of life. If you had dementia, which form of treatment would you like your carers to use? Physical force, pharmacological knock-out or lying to keep you safe?

THE CARE PROFILE

The objective of the SPECAL programme and process is to keep the feelings of the client in the *Green* zone by relating to their personal sense of reality. This 'reality' is different from present reality because many of the recent 'pictures' in their 'album' are missing. Learning from the client, we can build a Profile of what is important in their world. What the client sees as reality is probably based on a number of older pictures, especially from the time when the client was happy and productive. Relating to this out-of-date world through our communications with the client keeps them in a comfortable state, the *Green* zone.

The purpose of the client's Care Profile is to share with other carers what is important to the client's reality world. This is a summary of what you, as the main carer, have found to be the client's world. The key points, if written down as a list, are an invaluable tool for other carers, so they can also guide and keep the client comfortable, in the *Green* zone.

These are the main components of a Care Profile. They are the key points from the headings indicated above, very specifically for the individual client:

- *The Primary Theme.* The title of this with a summary of cue words, physical props and gestures. This is a key starting point.
- *The Health Theme.* Again, the title with catchphrase and key words. This should also be supported with props and gestures.
- *Departure Explanation.*

- *Absence Explanation.*
- *Presence Explanation.*
- *Altruistic Trigger.*
- *Most frequently asked questions* by client and most useful answers.

EXAMPLE OF A CARE PROFILE

The example given below is for Robert, the ex-RAF flying officer who was an aeroplane-spotting and birdwatching enthusiast.

- *The Primary Theme.* Ex-RAF flying, aeroplane-spotting and birdwatching enthusiast.
  Key words: RAF, air force, "Check who's flying in!"
  Props: pair of binoculars, 'Wings' on dressing gown pocket.
  Gesture: clenched fists in front of eyes, as if using binoculars.
- *The Health Theme.* Previous back problem. Recurrent malaria.
  Words: "Check if you're air-worthy." "Take care, avoid a prang." "Take care, don't want to be 'gone for a Burton' or have a bumpy landing."
  Prop: walking stick ready at hand.
  Gesture: rub hand on lower back (back ache).
- *Departure Explanation.*
  Words: "Pre-take off toilet visit." "Getting the gear ready."
  Gesture: hold nose and pull imaginary toilet chain.
- *Absence Explanation*
  Words: "Gone to get supplies/birdseed for feeders."
  Gesture: fingers of one hand pecking palm of other, i.e. bird-feeding.
- *Presence Explanation*
  Words: "Come to ask you about bird migration patterns."
  Gesture: pick up favourite Bird Book from the table.

- *Altruistic Trigger*
  Words: "Wait for instructions from control tower." "Possible emergency." "Crew have scrambled, wait for orders."
  Gesture: picking up phone and holding to ear.
- *Most frequent questions and appropriate replies.*
  Q. "When do we take off?"
  A. "As soon as the order comes."
  Q. "Where is Mavis?"
  A. "Getting the gear together."
  Q. "What's for supper?"
  A. "Something hot."

Alzheimer's disease and comfortable communications

Cardinal rules for SPECAL – a brief reminder

1. Don't ask questions.

2. Agree with everything they say.

3. Don't contradict, but endorse and encourage.

The following list takes the SPECAL principles a few steps further:

- Never ask questions, instead reminisce.
- Never argue, instead agree.
- Never reason, instead divert.
- Never shame, instead distract.
- Never lecture, instead reassure.
- Never say, "I told you," instead repeat.
- Never say, "You can't," instead say, "Shall we do..."
- Never demand, instead ask, "May we..."
- Never condescend, instead encourage.
- Never force, instead reinforce.

Note that the objective is not to distress but always to reassure the client.

Contented Dementia, as things progress

Unfortunately, there is usually a sad and difficult end-stage of dementia. Most of the above account about Contented Dementia and the SPECAL method, summarised from Oliver James' book, relates to the early and middle stages of dementia. Hopefully, by using this personalised method, the client will continue to have a long period of contented life. However, Peggy Garner admits that there is a serious end stage and she recommends that the primary carer and the client's family should prepare for this in advance.

There are two things that can be started at an early stage that will help carer and client for the serious end stage. The first is to gather, train and manage a care team who will help you or the primary carer look after the client. No matter how dedicated a carer is, ultimately he or she will need help to share the physical and psychological load. The second is to find the right care home to which the client will need to be admitted in the end stage. It may be a final phase which could be as short as a few days, but it could also be for years.

LEADING THE CARE TEAM

No matter how dedicated the main carer is, that person, and perhaps it is you, must recognise that there is a real danger of becoming isolated, burnt out and even demented.

A client needs to have a social structure for life: family, friends, neighbours, professionals and other contacts. They all have a role. Therefore, try to strengthen the social infrastructure of the client's life, and your own, as main carer. Often, family and friends like to help in small ways, but as team leader you will need to train and keep them motivated. It is a considerable but worthwhile task.[85]

First you need to educate everyone who is in contact with the client to avoid words and situations that can quickly hurt, alarm and take the client into a *Red* zone. Ask everyone to keep bad and negative news out of the way.

Teach the whole team about the SPECAL method. This is essential. The basis is understanding dementia from the point of view of the person with dementia.[86] Use the analogy of a photograph album for the memory: recent photographs, recent memories, seem to be missing but older pictures are still there, vivid and memorable. This enables carers to adapt their behaviour to take account of the dementia and manage it in a highly effective way. You will need to share with the whole team what is the client's Primary Theme and Care Profile. With a little training, probably a few people from the core team will be able to substitute for you.

Remember, try to avoid leaving the client alone with someone, especially a doctor or nurse, until you have briefed the person about the main SPECAL rules,[87] including the first, "Avoid asking questions." Also, share with health professionals the client's Health Theme.

Many people find visiting someone with dementia daunting, but it is important.[88]

PLANNING FOR A NURSING HOME

Every main carer should ask themselves the question, "When would it be safer for the client, and for everyone, if the client was transferred to full-time professional care?" The final pattern of illness varies and such a tipping point might come in different

---

[85] See the section entitled 'Build circles of support and join helpful networks' page 84.
[86] See the section entitled 'A patient-centred care for all those with dementia' on page 83.
[87] See page 154.
[88] See the section entitled 'Visiting someone with dementia' on page 102.

ways: "He almost set the house on fire," or, "She fell out of bed again and could not get up alone," or, "He 'escaped' from the house and got lost, again," or, "She kept me awake all night and I cannot go on without sleep," or, "He wants someone near him all the time, 24/7."

Penny Garner recommends that the main carer should not only consider this, but should select a suitable nursing home well before any client reaches the 'tipping point'. She sets out a series of sensible criteria of which the first is the willingness of the home to keep using the SPECAL method, which can be used to ease the transfer and ensure continuing comfortable care. Several potential homes should be visited that would suit the client and family, and the client's name placed on the waiting list, even if the point is never reached.

DECEPTION AND REALITY – DOES LOVING CARE TRUMP HARD TRUTH?

Penny Garner maintains that the objective of the SPECAL method is not to deceive, but to give comfort and confidence to the person with dementia, in the reality in which they live. To them, the situation of today is incomprehensible because of the lack of recent memory pictures that explain what is going on. Therefore, as carer you encourage them in believing in the old picture which they see clearly. You are speaking to their reality for the sake of their comfort and wellbeing. The method gives real care and comfort to the clients, the patients suffering from this dreadful, difficult and deadly disease. SPECAL is authentic, professional care and is fully justified.

Some people are opposed to basic aspects of the SPECAL technique. They say it involves speaking and living lies. It is helping the client to live in an imaginary false world. It may require a degree of subterfuge or deception, and replacing common sense with what Penny Garner called "SPECAL sense" which tries to understand the world from the perspective of the person with dementia. The reality for the client is based on their personal 'photo album' from years ago. By contrast, the present world is a world from which many of the recent pictures are missing.

The purpose of the SPECAL method is truly patient-centred care (PCC). It keeps a client comfortable by helping them live with the limited brain function they have. It encourages them to think that 'all is well' because they are reassured that they are living in an old reality, past experience, a time in which they were happy and in control; in fact, they are kept in that delusional state by the carers. They are kept safe in that state by the compassion and competence of the carers but this is a living lie. However, Penny argues that this is much better than being in the constant state of panic and anxiety of thinking, "My memory is going. I do not know how to cope. I am losing myself. Help!" Compassion trumps truth. It is legitimate 'post truth'!

In our personal experience, mine and that of my wife with early dementia, it is a matter of living in two worlds. There is the past, which at times seems clearer to her, and the present, which is real but infuriating and sometimes frightening because pieces of recent memory are missing.

In this situation, some but not all of the SPECAL techniques are relevant. For example, it is sensible not to ask any unnecessary or challenging questions, but it is not sensible to authenticate all statements she makes (SPECAL rules 1 and 3). When my wife says, "Where are my keys? I always leave them in my coat pocket," I don't simply 'authenticate' that, but it may be sensible to say, "Let us look on the hall table," because I saw them there a few minutes ago!

In an intelligent person who knows that he or she has early dementia, it may not be sensible or possible to apply the full SPECAL method. An example of this is Dr Jennifer Bute, who appreciates the benefits of SPECAL. She recognised her own dementia and does not deny it. She lives with it, sharing her experience with others, explaining what she is going through.

Similarly with my own wife; she is aware that she has dementia, but lives with it in confidence that she will be cared for and loved despite memory and functional limitations. I believe she shows spiritual serenity knowing that she is, and will be, loved by God and her family to the end. Fear and frustration appear to have been overcome by Christian confidence and composure.

In Lighter Mode: Lost, More Than the Car Keys

Several days ago, as I left a meeting, I desperately gave myself a personal search. I was looking for my keys. They were not in my pockets nor in my handbag. A quick search in the meeting room revealed nothing. Suddenly, I realised I must have left them in the car. Frantically, I headed for the car park.

My husband had often scolded me for leaving the keys in the ignition. My theory: in the ignition is the best place not to lose them. His theory: the car will be stolen.

As I scanned the car park, I came to a terrifying conclusion: his theory was right; the car park was empty. I immediately called the police. I gave them my location, described the car, confessed that I had left my keys in the car and it had been stolen.

Then I made the most difficult call of all.

"Hello, my love," I stammered. (I always call him "my love" in times like these.) "I left my keys in the car and it has been stolen."

There was a period of silence. I thought the call had disconnected, but then I heard his voice. He barked, "I dropped you off!"
Now it was my time to be silent. Embarrassed, I said, "Well, come and get me."

He retorted, "I will, as soon as I can convince this aggressive police officer that I have not stolen your car."

In Lighter Mode: Auto Hijack

An elderly lady did her shopping and went back to the car park. There she found four young men in the act of leaving with her vehicle. She dropped her shopping bags, drew her hand gun from her purse and screamed at the top of her lungs, "Get out of my car. I have a gun, and I know how to use it!" The four men didn't wait for a second threat. They got out and ran like mad.

The old lady, somewhat shaken, loaded her shopping into the car and got into the driver's seat. But her hands were shaking, and she could not get her key into the ignition. She tried and tried, and then she realised why. It was for the same reason she had wondered why there was a football, a Frisbee and a six-pack of beer beside the front seat.

A few minutes later, she found her own car parked five spaces farther down. She loaded her bags into the car and drove to the local police station to report her mistake. The sergeant to whom she told the story couldn't stop laughing. He pointed to the other end of the counter, where four pale men were reporting a carjacking by a mad, elderly woman described as white, less than five feet tall, with glasses, curly white hair, and carrying a large handgun.

This is a true account recorded in the Police Station Log of Sarasota, Florida, U.S.A. No charges were filed against the lady.

Chapter Ten

Care for the Carers

When a person in the family gradually gets dementia, it is often another family member who slowly becomes that person's carer. It has been called "the unexpected new career" and can become a full-time job. Gradually, you have to take over everything for them: healthcare, nourishment, social contacts, finances, the lot. You may not feel up to it yourself, either physically or psychologically. Friends, and even relatives, distance themselves.

Carer's burnout

Carer's burnout is a real possibility and can be fatal for both the carer and cared for!

Martha had been forgetful for some years, but when she was 75 things started to get really difficult. Her husband, Michael, who was nearly 80, had adjusted and coped well for two years. Progressively he took over the housework. Their daughter Milly, who lived at the far side of the country, visited after about a year and was horrified. The house was filthy, much of the food in the fridge was rotten, both parents had lost weight. Half-full bottles of pills implied that many doses had been missed. Martha's soiled clothes had accumulated and she had nothing clean to wear. She used to get up at night and wander so all doors had to be locked. Michael, who had been a meticulous man, was dishevelled, exhausted and burnt out from lack of sleep trying to stop Martha from harming herself. The couple were isolated; the family was far away, they were shunned by neighbours, and they were neglected by the public services, who believed Michael when he said they were "doing fine". In reality, the couple were in crisis. Milly realised that her father's valiant efforts to care for his wife meant that both her parents now needed care. The situation had progressed to serious double trouble.

Care for the carer and preventing burnout

While devotedly caring for a loved one with dementia, even the most loving personalities are buffeted by feelings of guilt, inadequacy, frustration, anger, stress, depression and insomnia. Take proper physical, psychological and spiritual care of yourself. This is vital or you cannot help your loved one well.

Caring for yourself is not an extra, it is not selfish; it is of core importance.

- *Take time for yourself every day* – even just 10 or 20 minutes.
  Do something that refreshes you: walk in the open air, listen to music, meditate, sleep. A few hours 'off duty' will help you to recharge your batteries. Reducing your stress will make you a better carer.
- *Know your limits.*
  Prepare for tasks, list them and pace yourself.
  You can't provide good care if you feel overwhelmed and stressed out. Learn when to say no. Set boundaries to protect yourself.
  If people offer to help, learn to say yes and make a list of things that people can help you with. Recognise that you cannot do everything yourself. Don't be proud.
- *Ask for help.*
  No one can take on all responsibilities for care alone. Discuss your needs with family and friends, explain how

others can help and tell them that their family member still needs company.

- *Make it a team effort.*
  Hold regular 'family meetings' to discuss any medical developments or new concerns or tasks, financial issues and your need for support. Include everyone who cares for your loved one, including paid helpers. Connect with more distant family members. Follow up any meeting with notes on sharing jobs and a calendar of tasks.
- *Stick to a daily or a weekly routine.*
  This can give a sense of security. You will feel in control and your loved one will know what to expect.
- *Join a support group.*
  Other carers understand your position best.
  Major charities have personnel to help: Alzheimer's Society, Carers UK and ageUK have support staff.
- *Some electronic devices can be helpful.*
  Timers and reminders can let you know when the next dose of a medicine is due. Pressure pads can alert you when your loved one has got out of bed or gone through a special door. There is a device that sends a message to a relative when the kettle is switched on in the morning. "Ah, she's up and making her first cuppa."
- *Let animals assist you.*
  Calm dogs, friendly cats, small birds and even fish can give purpose, occupational therapy and companionship, and make life more cheerful for everyone.
- *Turn on some music.*
  It can revive memories, spark smiles, start singing, clapping and stimulate shared fun moments for carer and the cared-for.
- *Try some simple art projects.*
  A simple art project can relieve stress. Colouring, painting or collage can relieve tension all round.

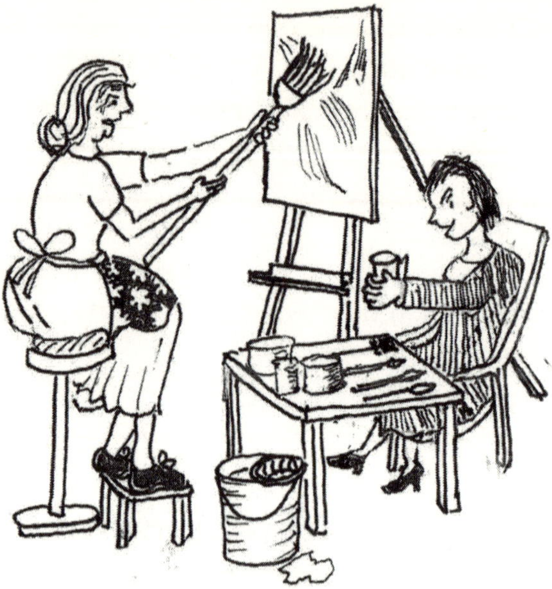

A painting or colouring project.
It doesn't have to be this ambitious.

Oh, one more thing… Paul wrote to his friends in Rome:

Don't burn out; keep yourselves fueled and aflame.
Be alert servants of the Master, cheerfully expectant.
Don't quit in hard times; pray all the harder.

Romans 12:11-12 (MSG)

A Poem for Carers and the Cared-For

Brother, sister, may I thank you,
Thanks for being Christ to me.
Thanks for all the love and care
On this lonely road with me.

When I feel so dull and stupid,
Friendly faces seem unknown,
Questions are for me a puzzle,
But when you're near, I'm not alone.

In my time of dark confusion
When all names and meanings go,
When my mind seems blank and barren
Then I need your love to know.

Once I'd work thro' each new question.
Things no longer make good sense.
Now I'm groping with my reason,
Leaves me with a feeling tense.

When I oft' repeat my questions,
Please be patient with my cries.
Often I don't recognise
That my memory's in demise.

When I was low, at sorrow's gate,
Living in a gloomy phase,
You 'minded me that life was great
So I'd relive my happy days.

Simple things I should remember,
From my brain they all depart.
If you sing the songs of childhood
Words and music flood my heart.

Your friendly chats at times confuse
And clever language can me scare,
But a gentle touch can warmth infuse
And a loving hug expresses care.

On well-known routes I lose my way,
And journeys make me anxious.
Perhaps my brain has gone astray,
But my soul is safe with Jesus.

Reference

A great source of information in UK is the charity Carers UK,
20 Great Dover Street, London SE1 4LX
General enquiries: 020 7378 4999, Email: *info@carersuk.org*
Advice line: 0808 808 7777

In Lighter Mode: Purposeful Endearments

An elderly lady was invited to an old friend's home for dinner one evening.

She was impressed by the way her friend, the hostess, preceded every request to her husband with endearing terms such as 'my love', 'darling', 'my dear', 'sweetheart', etc. The couple had been married almost sixty years, and clearly they were still very much in love.

While the husband was out of the room, the guest said to the hostess, "I think it's wonderful that after all these years, you still call your husband all those loving names."

Her elderly friend blinked her eyes. "The truth is," she replied, "I've forgotten his name and I'm scared to keep asking him; he's such a cranky old donkey!"

In Lighter Mode: The Value of the Written Word

An elderly couple are both having problems remembering things.

During a check-up, the doctor tells them that they're physically okay, but they should write things down to help them remember.

That evening, while watching TV, the old man gets up. "Want anything while I'm in the kitchen?" he asks.

"Will you get me some ice cream?"

"Sure."

"Don't you think you should write it down, so you can remember it?" she asks.

"No, I can remember it."

"Well, I'd like some strawberries on top, too. Maybe you should write it down so as not to forget it?"

He says, "I can remember that. You want a bowl of ice cream with strawberries."

"Oh, I'd also like whipped cream. I'm certain you'll forget; write it down!"

Irritated, he says, "I don't need to write it down; I can remember it! Ice cream with strawberries and whipped cream – I got it, OK?" Then he toddles into the kitchen.

After about 20 minutes, the old man returns and hands his wife a plate of bacon and eggs.

She stares at the plate for a moment and asks, "Where's my toast?"

Chapter Eleven

Prevent Dementia and Slow Its Progress

"Is it possible to prevent dementia?"

"When dementia occurs, is it possible to slow the progress of the disease?"

The answer to both questions is: *Yes,* to a significant extent, and *no,* not in everyone and not completely.

The mechanisms that cause the disease are still not fully known; there is no vaccine to prevent it and no 'magic bullet', no specific drug, to reverse the condition. Recent anti-amyloid drug trials failed to improve brain function. Therefore the importance of prevention has a new emphasis and urgency.[89]

We will begin with a review of the evidence about the causes and risk factors for dementia.

Lifestyle choices can decrease the incidence of dementia

This was demonstrated by Dr Peter Ellwood and colleagues in his classical longitudinal study in the Welsh town of Caerphilly. In 1979 he recruited 2,500 men aged 45-59 (about 90% of the men in that age group).

[89] LeCouteur D.G., Hunter S., Brayne C.; *Solanezumab and the amyloid hypothesis for Alzheimer's disease;* BMJ (2016); BMJ 2016;355:i6771.

He followed their health, morbidity and mortality with great care for three decades.[90]

He identified five healthy lifestyle behaviours:

- Not smoking.
- A low body weight – a BMI of less than 18. (BMI – body mass index – is weight in kilograms divided by the square of height in meters.)
- Regular exercise – at least half an hour of walking or equivalent exercise on 5 of 7 days a week.
- A diet low in fat but rich in fruit and vegetables.
- Alcohol consumption within accepted guidelines – 21 or less units each week.

Men who practised at least four of the five healthy behaviours had a 64% reduction in dementia or cognitive impairment. They also had a 67% reduction in heart attacks and strokes, a 73% reduction in diabetes and a 35% reduction in cancer.

These other matters are also of relevance as looking after the heart, the blood vessels, blood pressure and blood glucose are all relevant to looking after the brain. This is sound evidence of the significance of these factors in decreasing dementia. However, it does not guarantee that if you use all these practices you will never get Alzheimer's disease!

Other more recent studies have shown that healthy lifestyle factors, specifically the maintenance of a normal body weight, regular physical activity and a healthy diet, reduce brain shrinkage, and reduce sticky amyloid brain plaques and tau tangles which are found in the brains of many who die with Alzheimer's disease. Dr David Merrill and colleagues went further; they showed that it is possible to detect the influence of these lifestyle factors at a molecular level before the beginnings of

---

[90] Ellwood, P. et al.; *Healthy Lifestyles Reduce the Incidence of Chronic Diseases and Dementia: Evidence from the Caerphilly Cohort Study;* PLoS One (Dec 2013): 8(12): e81877. Published online. See also: *www.youtube.com/watch?v=U6Uj6K9MFKg*

serious memory problems. These simple lifestyle factors give some protection or "cognitive reserve" to the ageing brain. He concluded, "This work lends key insight into the ability of people to prevent Alzheimer's disease."[91]

Dr Clare Walton, research manager at Alzheimer's Society, said, "Regardless of how it works, the message is clear, there are steps people can take to keep their heads healthy as well as their hearts as they age."[92]

Risk factors for dementia

Now the thrust of recent research has swung to, "What are the risk factors for dementia and how can these be reduced?"

So, what is the evidence about risk factors and how can this information be used to reduce the onset or slow the progress of dementia?

In the largest international conference on research into dementia, held in London in 2017, the main emphasis and reports were on risk factors and ways in which the condition can be prevented. The additional risk factors for which there was evidence were hearing difficulties; sleep disturbance, especially from a degree of respiratory obstruction; psychological depression; and social isolation in later years. Early detection and corrective therapy is possible for most of these factors.[93]

Professor Gill Livingson, a leading presenter at the research conference, gave an optimistic challenge: "Acting now on dementia prevention, intervention and care will vastly improve

---

[91] Merrill, D.A. et al.; *Modifiable Risk Factors and Brain Positron Emission Tomography Measures of Amyloid and Tau in Nondemented Adults with Memory Complaints;* Am J Geriatr Psychiatry (Sep 2016): 24(9):729-37. doi: 10.1016/j.jagp.2016.05.007. Epub: 13 May 2016.

[92] Clare Walton; *Exercise can keep the mind young;* The Spectator (Health) 3 (May 2016). Clare Walton is Research Manager at Alzheimer's Society, UK.

[93] Wise, J.; *Dementia research focuses on prevention, as drugs fail to deliver;* BMJ 2017;358:13466.

living and dying for individuals with dementia and their families, and in doing so, will transform the future for society."[94]

Joseph Jebelli has recently reviewed the factors that fight against Alzheimer's disease.[95] He and many participants at the research conference concluded that all positive factors must be used and combined wherever possible to prevent onset, and delay progress, of this serious condition.

The proportion of dementia cases caused by genetic factors, and therefore not yet amenable to preventive measures, is possibly less than one third. Even in these people, healthy ways of living and positive activities may delay the start and slow the progress of dementia. Therefore, in conclusion, for the majority of those living with or without dementia, positive prevention measures are worthwhile. Lifestyle and other choices can significantly influence the progress and what life with dementia will be like.

The sections below describe interventions for which there is some evidence of benefit.

Look after your body

You will need the aid of your professional helpers with some things.

- *Keep your heart and blood vessels healthy.*
  Check blood pressure. A high blood pressure may be associated with damage to blood vessels, stress on the heart and poor blood supply to the brain. Avoid excess salt consumption; cut down your intake. If you have high blood pressure, use the effective medicines for this.
  Cholesterol levels can be checked. High HDL cholesterol is not significant, but raised LDL is associated with blockage of blood vessels in the heart and probably also the brain.

[94] Livingson G. et al.; *Prevention and management of dementia: a priority for public health;* Lancet (Jul 2017). *http://dx.doi.org/10.1016/S0140-6736(17)31363-6*

[95] J. Jebelli; *In pursuit of memory. The fight against Alzheimer's;* Hodder and Stoughton (London, 2017).

Both suitable diet and statin medication can lower high cholesterol.

Blocked or bleeding blood vessels in the brain cause damage and vascular dementia. Prompt treatment for stroke can limit damage.

- *Care for vision and hearing.*

  A person who does not see clearly or hear properly cannot respond or remember. This is so obvious; it is a literal and metaphorical 'no brainer', but it is easily neglected! Early detection of hearing loss and impaired vision are relatively easy and correction is possible. These deserve emphasis.
- *Protect the brain from injury in sports.*

  Avoid boxing or professional football heading. Reduce road accident trauma by wearing effective helmets and seat belts.
- *Deficiency of thyroxine, the hormone from the thyroid gland, and deficient levels of vitamins B12 and Folic acid can mimic dementia.*

  These have to be specifically tested for, but can be replaced.

MAKE DELIBERATE LIFESTYLE CHOICES

- *Exercise* appears to be the master key to health of body and brain. In a major recent analysis, there is good evidence that, "Physical exercise improved cognitive function in the over 50s, regardless of the cognitive status of participants."[96] To be most effective, the exercise should be for "a duration of 45-60 minutes per session" and at least moderate intensity of either or both "aerobic and resistance exercise", at least once and preferably several times a week. But lower intensity exercise is also valuable.

---

[96] Northey, J.M., et al.; *Exercise interventions for cognitive function in adults older than 50: a systematic review with meta-analysis;* Br J Sports Med (2017): 0:1–9. doi:10.1136/bjsports-2016-096587.

Moderate exercise in adults can not only help to avoid gradual reduction of brain size, but can actually improve cognitive function.

Regular exercise has been shown to increase brain activity. It has been shown to improve the connections – synapses – between nerve cells of the brain.

Exercise releases endorphins improving mood and fighting off stress and depression.

Exercise in groups, often with music, sometimes with a simple element of dance and co-ordination, improves motivation and adds an important social element.

> "Through regular physical exercise older people can increase their fitness level to that of an average person a decade younger. Evidence is growing that recovery of fitness improves cognitive ability and reduces the risk of dementia, not only in midlife but also in the 70s and 80s."[97]

- *Eat wisely and well, but not too much.* There is no single or even group of dietary constituents that can fully protect or cure a damaged brain. The best recommendation is a Mediterranean style of diet with plenty of fruit, vegetables, whole grains, nuts and some fish. Dark chocolate (high in coco) in modest amounts has some evidence to support it and can be the reward option. Eating together can add stimulation to pleasure.

  A wealthy country diet, high in animal fats and sugar, often served in too large portions, can contribute to obesity, one of the risk factors.

[97] McNally, S.; *Focus on physical activity can help avoid unnecessary social care;* BMJ (Oct 2017); 359:j4609; doi: 10.1136/bmj.j4609.

| *Try to keep your BMI*[98] *to less than 25.* |

- *Minimise alcohol intake.* There have been some conflicting reports about alcohol. However, a recent authoritative study indicates that even moderate alcohol consumption, drinking habits that many would consider 'normal', is associated with brain damage and cognitive decline. Those who drank very little or followed abstinence had least damage.[99]
- *Sleep* is important because during sleep some potential toxins are flushed from the brain. Inadequate quantity and particularly quality of sleep is important, but there is a wide variation in requirement from five to ten hours. A sound sleep is obviously more beneficial than restless sleep.
  A good night may depend on a good evening. Avoid heavy eating and drinking before retiring. Avoid stressful tasks and discussions, traumatic thoughts, horror movies and books before bed. Instead try to dwell on peaceful, positive matters to give restful sleep.
  There is evidence that people who have sleep apnoea, periods of a few seconds when they stop breathing during sleep, sometimes associated with snoring, are at greater risk of dementia. Usually this is in people who are overweight and have a thick neck. The first advice is to lose weight, avoid much alcohol, a heavy meal or sleeping pills just before going to bed. Referral to a Sleep Clinic for more detailed tests may be necessary.
- *Protect your mental health.* Depression, stress and anxiety can lead to memory loss. Often sympathetic care and better organisation of life timetable will decrease the issues that

---

[98] See definition of Body Mass Index (BMI) on page 181.

[99] Topiwala A., Allan C., Valkanova V. et al.; *Moderate alcohol consumption as risk factor for adverse brain outcomes and cognitive decline: longitudinal cohort study;* BMJ2017;357:j2353.
Killian, A.; *Alcohol consumption and brain health;* Editorial. BMJ (6 Jun 2017): 357; *https://doi.org/10.1136/bmj.j2645;* BMJ 2017;357:j2645.

cause the anxiety. Depression should not be considered as part of growing old. Professional help and medication should be sought by anyone with serious depression or when relatives notice significant change of mood.

Relaxation, meditation, mindfulness, and slow and deep breathing techniques can all be used to decrease stress and lower the body's stress hormones like cortisone. It is common knowledge that learning is less effective and judgement impaired in situations of stress.[100]

Older people should be encouraged to continue with any hobby, or indeed anything that stimulates curiosity. Continuing enquiry and stimulating activities are good.

An enriched environment stimulates an ageing brain; a garden with various colours and perfumes can evoke memories and give tranquillity.

- *Use your brain or lose it.* Consider your brain like a muscle; stop using it and its power will decline. To the contrary, learning increases synapses and neuronal circuitry.

  Seniors slip into habits. It is good to change your routine from time to time so that you do not do things automatically without thinking. Walk a different route, and change your timetable slightly to keep you thinking about times and seasons.

  Join in a memory club where there is stimulating company as well as simple quiz and word games. Do a daily crossword puzzle. Play Scrabble with a group of friends or even Online Scrabble. New and effective computer games specifically to engage the brains of older people are now becoming available.

  Challenge yourself; take up something that will stretch your brain: learn a new language, a new musical instrument, a new computer programme. Read out loud for 15 minutes daily: Shakespeare, the King James Bible.

[100] See page 126.

Challenges help to develop brain plasticity, new neurones and socialisation is believed to stimulate neural pathways. Keep curiosity alive. Be open to new ideas, experiences and inventions. It is said that 'curiosity killed the cat' but it may have the opposite effect on the ageing brain.

- *Socialise, participate in life.* Social connectivity, a sense of belonging, is very important. Relationships are part of being human; we are social animals and we must stay connected to stay stimulated. In isolation the brain withers. Loneliness and depression increase the risk of dementia by more than 50%. Several studies have confirmed a link between loneliness and dementia.
  People with friends and family have more mental and physical stimulation which boosts brain function. Those who live alone are at greater risk.
  Church congregations and other clubs, especially those with cross-generation contact, provide stimulation and socialisation. A faith that gives reassurance, hope and contentment is a buffer against anxiety, depression and isolation that are known risk factors for dementia.
  Music has a wonderful effect. A community choir combines music and socialisation. Sometimes those who have been mute can find voice, sing and smile!
- *Humour, mirth and laughter* are powerful tonics for the brain and spirit. Those living with dementia who can still read may enjoy simple comedies and even joke books. Some may have favourite TV situation comedies, play these old DVDs and laugh loudly, together with others when possible. Laughing together in company has multiple benefits to different parts of the brain.
- *Pets* can add a significant dimension to life. There is evidence that owning, caring for, feeding, grooming, touching and playing with animals and birds demands

attention and involvement, but it provides companionship and other benefits.[101]

MEDICATION HAS A LIMITED ROLE

There is currently no cure for dementia, but there are drugs that can help with some of the symptoms for some time. There are also medicines against some conditions that mimic or complicate dementia.[102]

Strengthen your spirit. Guard your heart.

Sometimes those who appear to have done all the best things do get progressive disease. At times the damage caused by dementia seems like the invasion of an evil power that has taken over your brain or the brain of your friend or beloved. Prepare yourself for such an attack with the spiritual weapons for combat. Paul was aware of malign forces and advised his friends to arm themselves with God-given weapons.

> *Finally, let the mighty strength of the Lord make you strong. Put on all the armour that God gives, so you can defend yourself against the devil's tricks. We are not fighting against humans. We are fighting against forces and authorities and against rulers of darkness and powers in the spiritual world. So put on all the armour that God gives. Then when that evil day comes, you will be able to defend yourself. And when the battle is over, you will still be standing firm.*
>
> *Ephesians 6:10-13 (CEV)*

---

[101] Gawande A, *Being Mortal; Illness, Medicine and What Matters in the End;* Profile Books Ltd. (London, 2014).
Cherniack, E.P., et al.; *The Benefit of Pets and Animal-Assisted Therapy to the Health of Older Individuals;* Current Gerontology and Geriatric Research (2014). doi: 10.1155/2014/623203. Published online.

[102] See the section entitled 'The role of medicines' on page 122.

Read the whole passage in Ephesians 6:10-18, and also read chapter 4 of this book.

References

Jebelli, J.; *In pursuit of memory. The fight against Alzheimer's;* Hodder and Stoughton (London, 2017)

Northey J. M. et al.; *Exercise interventions for cognitive function in adults older than 50: a systematic review with meta-analysis;* Br J Sports Med (2017);0:1–9; doi:10.1136/bjsports-2016-096587

In Lighter Mode: Senior Moments Poem

My forgetterer's getting better
But my rememberer is broke
To you that may seem funny
But, to me, that is no joke

For when I'm 'here' I'm wondering
If I really should be 'there'
And, when I try to think it through
I haven't got a prayer!

Oft' times I walk into a room,
Say, "What am I here for?"
I wrack my brain, but all in vain
A zero is my score

At times I put something away
Where it is safe, but gee!
The person it is safest from
Is generally me!

When shopping I may see someone,
Say, "Hi!" and have a chat,
Then, when the person walks away
I ask myself, "Who's that?"

Afterword

Since writing *Dementia: A Positive Response,* a large book has been published by Dr Dale Bredesen, an American dementia specialist with an attention-capturing title, *The End of Alzheimer's – The First Programme to Prevent and Reverse the Cognitive Decline of Dementia.*[103] The book demands some recognition and response.

What Bredesen means by the title is not clear. He admits that he has no 'silver bullet' against the disease and his regime is more of a shotgun approach against every possible risk factor.

He lists and gives much information about 36 risk factors for dementia and indicates how to detect each of these in an individual. He describes a battery of interventions to combat the risk factors and recommends applying *all* relevant interventions for an individual together in a protocol called ReCODE, which is short for 'Reversing COgnitive DEcline'. The total testing and intervention strategy would be very costly in time and money.

Many of the factors and interventions he lists are well known and are covered in *Dementia: A Positive Response.* Bredesen gives some striking case histories of patients who improved under the ReCODE protocol, but he gives no indication of the proportion of patients who improved. Unfortunately, there is no comment about prioritisation of risk factors or which interventions may be most useful and cost-effective. The book does not set out practical recommendations about how to manage and care for people with dementia in its different manifestations and stages.

---

[103] Dale Bredesen; *The End of Alzheimer's – The First Programme to Prevent and Reverse the Cognitive Decline of Dementia;* Vermillion, Penguin Random House Group (London, 2017).

Resources, Sources of Information, Help

The Dementia Guide. Living well after diagnosis; Alzheimer's Society (2017) This is a great resource, along with the website *www.alzheimers.org.uk*

ageUK has a good range of helpful booklets on many aspects of dementia and most of these are also available on their website.
www.ageuk.org.uk/health-wellbeing/conditions-illnesses/dementia/help-and-support/
Tavis House, 1-6 Tavistock Square, London WC1H 9NA

Carers UK, 20 Great Dover Street, London SE1 4LX
info@carersuk.org
General enquiries: 020 7378 4999
Advice line: 0808 808 7777

Helping to put the pieces together dementia information pack; Pilgrims' Friend Society (2013)
www.pilgrimsfriend.org.uk

Brain and Soul Boosting for Seniors; a workbook for Seniors and people with early dementia; Pilgrims' Friend Society (2016)
www.pilgrimsfriend.org.uk

Active Minds – activities and products for dementia; games, therapeutic activities, reminiscence activity kits, art activities, home care packs, personalised jigsaws, dementia clothing, etc.
www.active-minds.co.uk

Contact the Author

The author would be happy to receive comments or communications about this book at:

william.cutting@talktalk.net

Also by the Author

FACE THE FUTURE SERIES

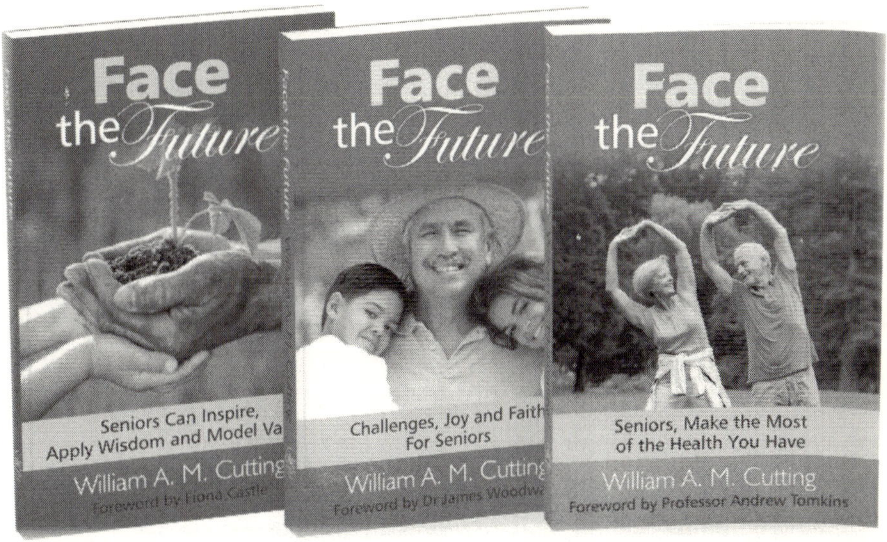

Face the Future 1
Seniors Can Inspire, Apply Wisdom and Model Values

ISBN 9781907509971

Face the Future 2
Challenges, Joy and Faith for Seniors

ISBN 9781910197110

Face the Future 3
Seniors, Make the Most of the Health You Have

ISBN 9781910197134

Books available from all good bookshops and from the publisher:

www.onwardsandupwards.org

Persiepone

Hymn 45

R 11

P 118

I've slipped from

love.

Hebrews 6

Acts 2 - Acts 19

Repent

Baptised

Believed

Great Joy

Holy Spirit

You cannot buy yourself a place in heaven.